LOVE AND FORGETTING

Love and Forgetting

A husband and wife's journey through dementia

JULIE MACFIE SOBOL & KEN SOBOL

Second Story Press

Library and Archives Canada Cataloguing in Publication

Sobol, Julie Macfie, 1936-, author
Love and forgetting : a husband and wife's journey through dementia /
Julie Macfie Sobol.

Issued in print and electronic formats.
ISBN 978-1-927583-18-0 (pbk.).—ISBN 978-1-927583-19-7 (epub)

1. Sobol, Ken—Health. 2. Sobol, Julie Macfie, 1936- —Marriage.
3. Lewy body dementia—Patients—Family relationships—Canada.
4. Lewy body dementia—Patients—Canada—Biography.
5. Authors, Canadian (English)—20th century—Biography. I. Title.

RC521.S67 2013   362.196'83   C2013-903873-6
                       C2013-903874-4

Edited by Nadiya Osmani and Carolyn Jackson
Copyedited by Kathryn White and Uzma Shakir
Designed by Melissa Kaita
Leaves © iStockphoto

Printed and bound in Canada

*Second Story Press gratefully acknowledges the support of the Ontario
Arts Council and the Canada Council for the Arts for our publishing
program. We acknowledge the financial support of the Government
of Canada through the Canada Book Fund.*

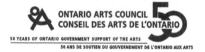

ONTARIO ARTS COUNCIL
CONSEIL DES ARTS DE L'ONTARIO
50 YEARS OF ONTARIO GOVERNMENT SUPPORT OF THE ARTS
50 ANS DE SOUTIEN DU GOUVERNEMENT DE L'ONTARIO AUX ARTS

 Canada Council   Conseil des Arts
for the Arts   du Canada

 MIX
Paper from
responsible sources
FSC   FSC® C004071
www.fsc.org

Published by
SECOND STORY PRESS
20 Maud Street, Suite 401
Toronto, ON M5V 2M5
www.secondstorypress.ca

To Lara Sanchez and Ximena Sanchez,
whose arrival on the scene
during the years covered in this book
brought us joy.

Love and forgetting might have carried them
A little further up the mountain side
With night so near, but not much further up.
　　　　　—Robert Frost, "Two Look at Two"

PROLOGUE

1959

Julie

I am in an upstairs room in Peters Hall, Oberlin College, Ohio, looking over Tappan Square. The class is Introspection and Observation: Philosophical Aspects of Psychoanalysis. A skinny, dark-haired boy whom I had seen around campus but never met came up to me after the bell rang. Was I headed for the library? he wanted to know. Yes, I was. Or I could be. We walked side-by-side to nearby Carnegie Library and ended up studying together all afternoon. Before we headed off to our dorms to get ready for dinner, I had agreed to a date the following Saturday.

That was the beginning of more than a beautiful friendship. On our first date, as we danced to a recording of "Serenade in Blue" in the rec center's darkened lounge, he recited a detailed history of the Six Tribes of the Iroquois

Confederacy in my ear. This was a new, and endearing, approach to courtship. I'd endured too many evenings with sweet but tongue-tied boys whose conversational skills were limited to asking if I liked my classes this year before sinking into awkward silence. How could I not be interested?

Ken was never at a loss for words back then. History—any kind of history—was a favorite topic; I'd learned that on our first date. But he had other things he wanted to talk about—for instance, how very different Europe was from Ohio. Ken had returned to the United States just days before the fall semester started and now, six months later, he was still full of stories about that year of discovery. We spent a lot of time talking in the library's smoke-filled student lounge. After he'd found matches and lit up our Salem cigarettes—a ritual of the era—I would put down my textbook and listen to his tales of hitchhiking through Spain, debating politics *sur les ponts de Paris*, and taking in brilliant sociology lectures at the London School of Economics.

Eventually, when we left Europe behind and moved on to other subjects, I was surprised and pleased to find that Ken, like me, read a lot of poetry. He, in turn, was only mildly indignant when he found out that, in addition to being familiar with poets past and present, I knew a lot of poems by heart and could always come up with quotations in defense of my opinions. Though I enjoy listening to a good talker, I also like to talk.

Still, I was secretly pleased when he took to telling his friends in mock amazement, "Can you believe it? I'm dating a girl who knows more poetry than I do. Amazing." (That was how boys talked back in 1959. It's hard now for me to believe

2

that we were only a couple of years away from Betty Friedan, bra burning, and Take-Back-the-Night marches.)

When did we first know we were becoming seriously involved? Maybe it was the spring weekend when Ken used some pretext to talk his mother into letting him borrow her car to drive us to New York. We spent two days exploring Manhattan and two nights sharing a single room in Hotel Edison.

Maybe we knew even earlier than that: the night Ken walked me back to the dorm after studying for mid-semester exams. That morning, one of the spring storms that every once in awhile blow inland from Lake Erie had covered the campus with a foot of snow and caused the temperature to plummet. The sidewalks were icy and treacherous, and suddenly my feet flew out from under me. I landed in a huge drift, my books and papers scattering all around. Ken immediately "slipped" too, and crashed down on top of me. We filled the icy night air with peals of laughter for no reason beyond the sheer enjoyment of the moment; only the bulky limestone buildings keeping us company, their sharp angles softened by the whiteness.

So many snowfalls since then, in so many different settings.

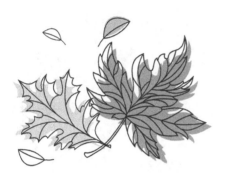

Part I

Leaving the Fields and Trees

CHAPTER 1

Julie

Spring, 2002—optimistic tulips push their way up through the last grimy traces of winter. Some forty-three years after our first meeting, Ken and I were living deep in rural Ontario. Overall I prefer city life to the country (previous stops in our nomadic life together had included stays in New York, London, Los Angeles, Cleveland, Montreal, and Toronto), but I've never regretted those years in the country: eight of them in a back-road log cabin halfway between the big cities of Montreal and Ottawa; then six years in a modern bungalow with a distant view of Lake Erie outside the kitchen window.

In both places, our involvement with local politics had led to some warm friendships (and some not so warm, but always interesting). Living in relative isolation had made us self-dependent and cognizant of ourselves as a part—a very small part—of the natural world. The nearby fields and woodlots, each with its own shape and microclimate, had become a familiar landscape in our shared world.

But—a *big* but—lately my mind was turning more and more toward Toronto. I could tell that even Ken, who always claimed to be a country boy at heart despite a childhood spent in Cleveland Heights, Ohio, was starting to feel the pull of city life. We needed more people around us; it was as simple as that. I would miss the fields and trees, but as we pulled up stakes and pointed the car eastward, I knew we were saying good-bye to the country for good.

By early summer, we were resettled in Toronto's Little Italy, with its crowded sidewalks, bicycles, outdoor cafes, and people galore. It was wonderful to be closer to our grandchildren and within a short walk of bookstores, museums, and even one of the few remaining neighborhood movie theaters. However, during one of our first expeditions out to see a play at Harbourfront, Ken became panicky. "We'll have to leave at the intermission," he whispered in the dark theater. "There's no chance of getting a taxi, and we shouldn't be walking around down here at this late hour."

Could he be serious? In danger at Queens Quay? That was ridiculous! When I pointed out that the theater was located on the top floor of a busy restaurant/shopping concourse, and that after the final act we were sure to find a whole fleet of cabs hungry for fares, he relented. But this was a guy who used to walk home through Brooklyn's dark, deserted streets in the early morning hours without a second thought.

What on earth was going on?

During the last few years in the country, there had been hints of trouble: a sudden dislike of crowds, problems communicating over the phone, bouts of irritability that came and went like the weather. We blamed it all on ageing, on the children living (at that point) far away, on a couple of long-time friendships ending, on the many hours of work we were putting in on our second book collaboration, *Lake Erie: A Pictorial History*. But these were a natural part of life, which up to now I thought we had been weathering pretty well. The theater panic was harder to explain away.

Over the next year other behavioral quirks made their appearance. One night I was awakened out of a sound sleep by a whoosh of air. In the dim light from the hall, I could make out blankets being swirled above my head, one after the other, as Ken experimented with various combinations of bed coverings.

"What's going on?" I asked.

"I can't get the damn covers right!"

There were a few more tries—quilt and blanket, two blankets, quilt by itself—before he found what he judged to be a satisfactory combination. At which point, one of us went right back to sleep and the other watched the sun rise as she drank her very early morning coffee and waited for the newspaper to be delivered.

The blanket issue became an obsession for Ken, so much so that though neither of us much likes shopping, we ventured out to one of those piled-high linen emporiums that offer bed coverings in every possible color, size, style, and weight. The lightweight duvet that Ken picked out solved the problem for the time being. And that was a relief.

But now the violent nightmares that had occasionally troubled him in the past became more frequent. During the worst of them, he would kick out in his sleep, thrash his arms around, shout out in loud defiance of his pursuers. I quickly learned not to grab his wrists when he was having one of these episodes; any touch could be interpreted as a threat. From deep within one dream, he landed a left hook on the side of my head. The blow didn't hurt, but he was deeply distressed to have done such a thing, even unintentionally.

And then, out of nowhere, there were the inexplicable sideways shifts in logic. The Sheets-on-the-Bed episode stands out in my mind. After transferring a load of wet clothes into the basement dryer one morning, I asked if he would bring down some linens from our room. He headed upstairs.

"There aren't any sheets," he reported cheerfully.

"Yes, of course there are. On the bed. Did you look?"

"Yes, I did. And *no*, there aren't."

We trudged back upstairs and stood side-by-side looking down at the mattress. He had a point, in a way. But "in a way" is very much the operative phrase. There certainly were no sheets hugging the mattress; I had stripped the bed earlier. They were rolled up into a large ball that was sitting on top of the mattress. When I pointed to it, Ken didn't react. He didn't laugh or look mildly foolish, as you would normally expect. He just picked up the sheets and, without a word, turned and headed back downstairs.

I also couldn't count the number of times over the last few weeks that he had become alarmed over losing his wallet, keys, or gloves. (None of those were really lost; they just weren't in the places he had looked.) And I had become aware of a slight tremor in his hands and an unnerving new habit of staring at me coldly (or so it seemed), not even blinking during conversations. A couple of times, when I asked if anything was bothering him, he insisted, "No, nothing at all. I have a good life. No complaints."

The tipping point came when Jane, our youngest daughter, dropped by. She studied Ken thoughtfully as he walked into the living room, then asked, "Dad, why are you shuffling around like that?" *Shuffling. That was the word!* Though I had noticed something different about his walk, it took the younger generation to bring that new quirk to the front of my mind. The slightest confirmation of something amiss can make a big difference; this first unsolicited acknowledgment from someone else of Ken's changed condition was so powerful that from that point on, as he grew more silent and moody with each day, I made sure to be more observant of his changes.

On the morning he confided in me his only-half-joking fear about the possibility of Alzheimer's, I didn't tell him that my thoughts were running in the same direction; but the next time I was at the library, I waited until a computer was free and looked through the long list of books on the condition. Selecting a couple of volumes from the shelf, I found a free seat, and began reading.

Mood swings were listed as a symptom. So were withdrawal from social events, misplacing things, difficulty with basic household tasks, and general forgetfulness about the recent past. To the first three, I could answer a definite "yes"—that was worrisome. But the last two, which appeared to be most typical of the disease, I put as "maybes." We're all forgetful as we grow older, but Ken hadn't yet put the ice cream in the oven or tossed the used cutlery in the garbage. And I hadn't noticed him forgetting the names of neighbors or the details of recent events.

I left the library somewhat reassured. Still, all these behavioral quirks—each one of them small enough by itself—were beginning to take on a critical mass. Since Ken was overdue for a checkup anyway, I talked him into seeing our family physician, Dr. Nguyen. After listening to his worries, the doctor was concerned enough to refer him to a neurologist.

On Ken's return from his visit to the specialist in October of 2006, his expression was hard to read. Disbelief? Bafflement? Plain-old fear? He slumped down onto the sofa. "That quack says I probably have Parkinson's disease," he said. "At least that's what I think he told me—he was a little hard to follow. I'm supposed to come back in six months." I also sat down, hard. We'd dealt with our share of illness over the decades, but somehow neither of us had contemplated the possibility of a neurological disease. Nor did we have much idea of what this one might involve.

We tried to be philosophical. We hugged, talked it over, and agreed to face the future with as much fortitude as we could muster. And there was a kind of comfort in at least having a name to put to his strange assortment of symptoms.

"Of course it's only a 'probable,'" we reminded each other, wishing all the while that the diagnosis had been clearer. "For Christ's sake," Ken ranted, "a doctor ought to know that uncertainty is the hardest thing of all to live with. That fact of life should rate at least a brief lecture in first-year med school! At least."

Our vaunted fortitude would soon be tested. Waiting in the wings was another "probable," though this one had nothing to do with anything neurological. Just before Christmas, an ominous Prostate-Specific Antigen (PSA) test was followed by a biopsy and then a command appearance at the urology clinic. "The good news is that prostate cancer is treatable," a grave-looking urologist reassured us. "And it's curable." That sounded good, but even better, I wanted to tell him, would have been hearing that the lab had made a mistake—that we were home free.

Four months later, Ken returned to the neurologist for a second assessment, expecting to hear confirmation of the original diagnosis. Instead, he was told that it was still too soon to tell and that he should come back in six more months. Without much trouble, we pushed aside thoughts of Parkinson's to make room for our concern about the upcoming series of radiation treatments scheduled for early June. Cancer worries trumped the neurological: Ken had been successfully treated for thyroid cancer eight years earlier, and I couldn't help wondering if that was related to the new cancer diagnosis.

My medical vocabulary expanded exponentially as I read my way through the handful of acronym-sprinkled booklets Ken brought home from the cancer hospital. (One of these directed you to a short animated film an acquaintance nicknamed "Your Friend, the Prostate.") Despite all the preparation, a new crisis—an agonizing urinary blockage—arose within hours of Ken's first treatment at the radiology clinic.

Before he knew it, he was in a hospital bed being prepped for a transurethral resection of the prostate, or "TURP" for short. "This procedure," the urologist cheerfully explained as he made quick little sketches on a scrap of paper, "is a simple dredging out of the urethra—really nothing to get alarmed about." As he described it, the process was more or less along the same lines as cleaning out a stuffed drain with a roto-rooter. Noticing our silence, he glanced up at Ken and quickly added, "And, it will be done under a very strong local anesthetic."

Sure enough, the TURP, performed on a mid-June morning, went so well that afterward in his room, I found Ken cracking jokes with his two roommates...relief all round. But by the next morning, when I phoned to ask how the night had gone, his mood had changed. His voice was subdued, not like him at all. He sounded strangely tentative, even confused.

"What city are you in, anyway?" he asked. "For some reason I keep thinking you're in Montreal."

Twenty years had passed since our last sojourn in *la belle province*; Ken knew that. And though typically his conversation is full of wry comments, I sensed he wasn't joking. Something was wrong—very wrong.

"Toronto," I told him. "I'm in Toronto; we both are."

No reply.

That evening, when Jane stopped by with her three-year-old daughter to ask how I was doing, I tried to answer but couldn't find the words to frame a reply, could only burst into tears as Ximena stared wide-eyed at the sight of Grandma losing it, falling to pieces against the kitchen table.

CHAPTER 2

Ken

I'm in the hospital. The TURP, I thought, had gone so smoothly that I decided to relax and take advantage of my recovery time. The presence of my two roommates, both about my age (I had celebrated my seventieth birthday on March 10), and both remarkably cheerful men, had a calming effect. The hours passed more quickly than they usually do in such circumstances until I crashed head first into what I can only describe as the classic "bad trip."

Bad trips. Remember those? This was a very, *very* bad trip. One in which my eyes popped open like cartoon moons to reveal an assortment of elderly jalopies herky-jerking their way through what seemed to be a reenactment of the opening scenes of Antonioni's film *Blow-Up*. One after another of these wrecks screeched to a halt at the door to the emergency room to disgorge dozens of passengers. I tried frantically to catch the attention of one of the strangely overdressed, giggling night nurses who regularly strolled by to check on us; but no one, to my surprise and annoyance, paid any attention. They persisted in dashing in and out, whooping and hollering as they disappeared behind a series of Chinese screens, where they were apparently holding a fancy-dress party.

I turned to look for my fellow inmates, but their beds were empty. I felt totally, terrifyingly alone, catapulted into a world I didn't understand, able to catch only tantalizing glimpses of nurses in elaborate, expensive gowns and doctors wearing hobo costumes as loud bursts of laughter and party noise drifted out from behind the screens.

Hours, or what seemed like hours, later I woke to see my son John walking toward me down the hallway. John told me later he hadn't been able to make head nor tail of what I had confided to him on the way home.

Julie
The operation was a minor one—Ken should have bounced right back, yet during the first days after his return, he just sat for hours in his favorite armchair, reading the paper or staring out the bay window at passersby.

John glanced over at him one evening during a visit from Ottawa. "Dad, where *are* you right now?" he asked.

Ken looked up, startled, then with an obvious effort replied, "Here, John. I'm right here. It's fine."

But it wasn't fine.

One night not long after, I woke to the sound of him moving around in the bedroom and then the back door closing quietly. I glanced at the clock: 4 a.m. *Help!* Ken had never before disappeared in the middle of the night without explanation. What should I do? He wasn't a kid, I reminded myself; he was perfectly capable of taking care of himself.

Did I believe that? I had to. Still, it was a relief, about half an hour later, to hear his key in the lock. I hurried to meet him at the door.

"Thank goodness you're here," Ken said. He gave me a hug, yawned, and mumbled something about "another one of those bad dreams." He glanced at me, then looked away. "You know, like the ones in the hospital…nothing, really… It's okay. I just need some sleep."

I phoned the urologist's office in the morning. A cheerful voice reassured me, "Nothing so unusual about this sort of stuff after an operation, Mrs. Sobol. It's probably the anesthetic. A few patients continue to have hallucinations at home, even after a couple of weeks. Don't worry."

I couldn't be quite that casual, having seen the look on Ken's face the night before. And our three kids, who had watched their dad sail through three previous surgeries— including the one for thyroid cancer—with no untoward side effects, felt the same way.

After a family lunch one warm Sunday afternoon, while Ken napped, I found myself in the living room of our older daughter, Corry, and her husband, Greg. Also present were Jane and our eldest, John. The five of us stared at each other, wondering how to start the conversation we knew we had to have.

There was an unspoken irony in the timing of this unusual get-together: the third Sunday in June, Father's Day. How weird to have a family meeting on this of all days without Ken here in person, full of opinions! The whole thing felt like betrayal: Ken wasn't the sort of dad who fades into the background after the children are grown, with kids of their own. He had always taken the job of parenting seriously, and perhaps the more so because his own childhood had been less than ideal. In fact, he hadn't spoken with his own parents for years.

Ken wrote about his early life in this excerpt from an unpublished 1983 biography.

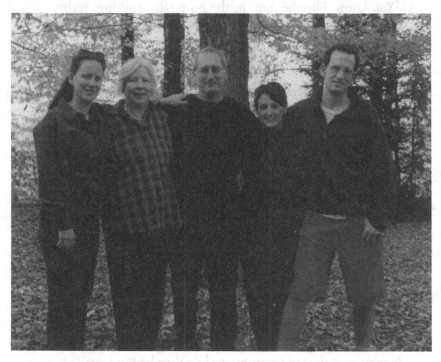

The Sobol family in carefree days, 1996: Jane, Julie, Ken, Corry, and John.

"I spent my first seventeen years in Cleveland Heights, Ohio, then an upper-middle-class suburb that not only boasted the traditional mid-western debilities of insularity and small-mindedness, but also a rigid ghetto clannishness. At the time, I didn't quite know that I hated it, but I was always conscious of being a misfit. What I remember most from my childhood is a gnawing loneliness and sense of always behaving wrongly no matter how hard I tried to conform. Many people who knew me would have said that I had never tried, but that's wrong; it's true that I was naturally rebellious, but I tried like hell.

"The central animating force of my parents' lives was fear of the outside world, and consequently they devoted a great deal of their time trying to manipulate their environment. As I was the main unpredictable variable in their existence, they worked me over night and day from early childhood on. The worst part was that they operated as a team: I could never appeal to one of them for relief from unfair judgment. And they succeeded in instilling in me a lot of their unease with the world.

"Life wasn't entirely dismal. I wasn't Oliver Twist, after all; the material comforts were always there. I had a good sense of humor, a strong imagination, and an endless supply of arrogance, so I struggled through without having my spirit entirely destroyed. Early on I looked for ways of getting away. Some days

I would just pack a lunch, get on my bike, ride thirty miles out into the Ohio countryside, and spend the day poking around. When I got older, I began hitch-hiking two or three times a year to New York City where I would hang around Washington Square or try to sneak into the jazz bars.

"Europe changed everything. I got off the boat at Cherbourg, France, in the summer of 1957 and took a train to Paris. (I hadn't memorized Hemingway, Fitzgerald, cummings, and the like for nothing.) During that year abroad, for the first time in my life, I made real friends, some of whom remain close to today. Many of them were Canadian, which would ultimately result in our immigrating to that country."

Our first impromptu visit to Canada had taken place in the summer of 1961, just three years after Ken's return from his European road to Damascus. He had announced one day that we were going to drive up to Toronto from Cleveland and look up some of the Canadians he had met in Europe. "You've heard me talk of Rick Arnold," he explained. "We lived in the same student boarding house." Yes, by now I knew those stories by heart; I'd heard them often enough. I knew Rick had married a girl named Veronica and brought his north-of-England bride back to Toronto. I was curious to meet the pair.

In those days, we scorned such bourgeois notions as phoning ahead. We shouldn't have been surprised, then, when we arrived at the Arnolds' address and found out they were away.

That didn't stop us from being illogically indignant; we only cheered up after it occurred to us that we didn't have to waste the opportunity to explore this strange just-over-the-border country, a place where most people spoke English (Montreal at that point was still far in the future) and yet where there were so many small differences, from the taste of the beer to the vari-colored money and the habit of slathering both butter and mayonnaise on their BLT sandwiches.

We headed deep into the countryside, driving for hours in a vaguely north direction, at one point pulling up in front of a small structure with a sign reading "Home of Artist Tom Thomson." Evidently, Tom was a big name in these parts and with good reason: the small landscapes on the walls were painted with color and conviction—you couldn't stop looking at them. In fact, we enjoyed exploring the area so much that we decided to look for a place to stay over for the night. "In for a penny, in for a pound." When the proprietors of our small motel pointed out a poster advertising a square dance in the village that same night, we completed our rural odyssey by do-sa-do-ing the night away with friendly locals.

Those twenty-four hours in Canada made a deep impression on us. We arrived in Toronto as landed immigrants in 1974. Certain details stand out from those early days: the pale complexions of the teenage waitresses at the restaurant stop on Highway 401, the beery British-working-man feel of the downtown bar where we stopped to ask directions, neighbors with exotic names like Vanessa and Basil and Clive. And the hairdresser at the College Street Hudson's Bay store who, when I mentioned in passing that I was a new arrival, put down his blow-dryer and demanded in an astonished voice, "Why on earth would you leave the States and come up here?"

His question demanded an answer. To my surprise I found myself telling him that sanity was undervalued as a national virtue (a thought I had never before expressed or even formulated, but as I said the words I found I meant them). The stylist gave me a look that seemed to say he didn't think I possessed much of that virtue myself.

"What do you mean?" he asked.

"Well…" I had to think. "Universal health care, for one example. It just makes sense, doesn't it?"

This was something else I was dimly aware of in those first weeks, though as with the sanity comment I hadn't ever articulated it—the wonderfully inclusive discovery that everyone, including the handcuffed convict who not long after our arrival sat across from me in a hospital waiting room, shared access to the same level of medical care. Health is a language universally spoken. After mulling over the thought, my hairdresser picked up the blow-dryer, nodded in agreement, and got back to work.

Yet now here I sat in that same city, more than three decades later, baffled as to what my next step should be. Finding the right specialist for Ken's mystery disease was proving to be a challenge, and without a clear diagnosis we were at a dead end.

Still, I was touched—once the conversation with our kids got past a somewhat disjointed opening—by their expressions of affection for their father and their level of support for me. When someone suggested checking out what our family doctor might say, and after John agreed to come along, I promised to call the next morning for an appointment. It felt good to determine any action, no matter how small.

Dr. Nguyen, when we arrived at his busy office, listened sympathetically to our story, but in the end had no suggestion beyond keeping calm while waiting for the neurologist's ultimate assessment. "At least he heard us out," I told John on our walk back to the apartment, "and it probably wasn't bad advice."

During the next few weeks, as Ken rested up in preparation for a second round of radiation therapy, I made a point of keeping busy and tried to bide my time. But it was hard. So many questions, so few answers. Even just formulating the questions was a challenge. Everything I read online about Parkinson's disease dealt exclusively with physical symptoms. Ken's palsy had increased slightly, which was worrisome, and there was that odd shuffling gait, but thankfully he showed no sign of being headed for a wheelchair any time soon. It was the other stuff that scared me: his moodiness, sudden obsessions, night terrors, and anxiety over such non-issues as finding a taxi. A brochure I had picked up mentioned hallucinations as a rare, unlikely symptom and devoted a short paragraph to "fluctuating cognition" but didn't go into any detail.

I was baffled; you can't force a diagnosis on a set of symptoms no matter how hard you try. Perhaps worst of all was the fact that no one outside the family noticed anything odd about Ken's behavior. Could it be that I was the one hallucinating? Some of the self-doubt ceased when one day a woman from a house across the street, going about her daily job of sweeping a stray leaf from her already immaculate front walk, waved me over. She demanded that I tell her why Ken had stopped acknowledging her greeting in his usual friendly way. "Your husband is not well, I think?" she said. I stammered out a noncommittal reply, though I actually welcomed my neighbor's Jane Jacobs–style view of herself as community watchdog; we could use more of that sort of thing in our cities. What some might interpret as nosiness I took to be concern.

After that encounter, I was better prepared when another neighbor, one with whom we shared a laneway and whom I had gotten to know as a friend, raised the same issue. Nancy listened intently as I gave her a quick rundown of the possible Parkinson's diagnosis and the fact that the radiation treatments had not gone well. She patted my arm and said, "I'm so, so sorry to hear about Ken's troubles."

These frank expressions of concern helped keep me going during that difficult summer. For now we were waiting for two things: the continuation of the radiation treatments after a break of several weeks and a conclusive (or so we hoped) diagnosis from Ken's neurologist.

CHAPTER 3

Julie

In late July, our family doctor offered up his cottage for a few days of R&R, and we jumped at the chance. We had been missing our friends the fields and trees and, with Ken scheduled to start radiation the next week, we needed this chance to get away. We packed our bags and headed north.

Somewhere near Collingwood, we pulled over and parked under some willows growing along Georgian Bay. We sat together on a couple of huge boulders, listening to the silence and staring out across the bright stretch of water. After an hour or so of idly watching the cold waves splash up against the granite, we jumped back in the car and drove inland, ending our journey high up in the green hills that parallel the lake. Blood tests and x-ray machines slowly faded from my mind as we breathed in the fresh country air.

In town that evening, I pushed open the door of the local Chinese restaurant and was greeted by the sight of Elvis, strangely thin and alive and dressed entirely in blue Lycra. The King rushed forward to shake our hands and, in a deep voice with a pronounced Australian accent, welcomed us. He was here in Collingwood, he informed us in his best Presleyan tones, for the largest Elvis gathering in Canada, an event that we should not fail to attend. We took his advice, scooping up the last available tickets for the gala competition.

There were some good musicians on the crowded roster in the ornate three-hundred-seat theater. Between them, the Elvis impersonators covered the King's entire repertoire, with only a few repeats of old favorites such as "Heartbreak Hotel" and "Hound Dog." We, like the rest of the enthusiastic crowd, enjoyed every minute of the nostalgic rock'n'roll evening. By the time we were back in our borrowed cottage, I felt refreshed.

Later, as we sat reading together, Ken cleared his throat and asked casually, "Is there anyone else staying in this place except for us?"

I put down my paper slowly. What a strange question! The modern, one-story, white-painted structure, part of a brand new cottage community, was not a likely spot for intruders. Or ghosts.

"No, just us," I told him. "Other people stay here sometimes, but right now it's just us."

"Funny, I keep thinking there's a bunch of other people."

I glanced around. *No, nobody else.*

Back in Toronto, the radiation treatments began where they had left off, and this time everything went well. We quickly settled into a five-days-on, two-days-off routine. One hot, smoggy Saturday, as we relaxed at a table outside a local coffee shop, Ken suddenly posed another of his mysterious questions.

"Have you ever experienced any floaters?"

A few years back, wiggly flashes of light had started moving across my field of vision from time to time. The doctor had called these "floaters" and told me not to worry; they would go away—which they had. But Ken shook his head when I described that phenomenon. "That's not it. Nothing like that."

"Okay. Well…can you describe what you mean, then? Just a few details," I said.

He thought for a moment. "It's like I'm seeing the same scene twice." He paused for a sip of coffee. "I mean, like something briefly repeated, the same but different."

I told him I didn't remember ever seeing anything like that.

He continued to look thoughtful. "Maybe I'll go have my eyes checked out."

However, when Ken went to the optometrist for a complete examination, the doctor just said he couldn't find anything to fret about.

During the final week of treatments in September, Ken and I were busy preparing to move into a sunny, new, high-ceilinged apartment. Though the place was only four blocks away from our previous one, it was worlds away in terms of the upheaval it would cause in our lives. As I've said, we were nomadic types who had moved many times—twenty, by an actual count made one day when we had nothing better to do. Another encounter with a moving van shouldn't be a big deal. Right?

Wrong! We didn't know it at the time, but you should give careful thought to the timing of any major changes if you think someone in the family is showing early signs of dementia.

Ken

I didn't have cataracts, or any other discernible eye problems, according to the optometrist. That was good, I guess. But as I walked home after the appointment, I was still worried. If the eye examination hadn't turned up anything, then what was causing all these strange visions? With this disease, whatever it might be, there seemed to be no easy answers.

Moving day was October 1, 2007. When I got up the first night at the new place to use the washroom, I was startled to find that the stacks of boxes, floor lamps, and other scattered leftovers from the move were providing material for new kinds of bizarre shapes. The forms were back again the next night. In fact, it got so that virtually every evening I would find waiting for me outside the bedroom door a troupe of odd, inexplicable creatures doing their best to shake my grip on reality.

These were not like the alarming nighttime apparitions I'd seen in the hospital after the TURP procedure. The new ones came in two basic guises: animals of various sorts—mostly small, scuttering creatures—and tall, thin types. Sometimes they ignored me. Sometimes, but only if I turned toward them and stared, they became animated. Then, for example, the low rectangular radiator in the hallway might suddenly convert itself into a small sheep; a cluster of scarves on the coat hook might become a high fashion hat; an Inuit print could spring to life as a circle of wolves following me with their eyes. (A litho resembling such a wolf scene hangs on the wall of our home office.) Some of the more feminine figures, if that is the proper designation for them, carried what appeared to be small creatures in their arms.

At first, I freaked. No surprise there. But then I noticed that whenever I approached them, they would immediately rise and move off in slow motion down the hallway, or simply disintegrate on the spot, before reforming into normal lamps, jackets, and whatever other objects in the darkness had led me to imagine their existence.

On the nights that followed, some of the forms even entered our bedroom and then at times, I had to waken Julie to make sure they went away. (Not that she ever saw them, of course, but her voice was reassuring to me and commanding to the apparitions.) Ultimately, it seemed clear to me they meant no harm nor presented any real danger. All the same, when I later came across a reference book that called them "benign visions," I was relieved.

I rarely got a glimpse of the hall dwellers' faces; I wasn't even sure they had any. They never spoke, and except for one accidental instance, they always managed to fade away before I made physical contact. The incident where I touched one took place as I came out of the bathroom one evening and tripped on something (a shoe, I think), losing my balance. As I thrust out my arm toward the wall to catch myself, so did a vaguely alpaca-like creature. We met and touched at a corner—Julie's terrycloth bathrobe and my shaggy Irish wool sweater hanging on the coat rack. The creature and I both sprang back in alarm. When I looked again it had disappeared, fading into the woodwork.

I didn't know what to make of this tactile experience; I still don't. But as time passed, I grew so accustomed to the apparitions that I began looking forward, albeit in a slightly uneasy way, to seeing what form they would take each night.

Then there were those other apparitions, the ones that could come at any time and that manifested themselves not as things I see, but as things watching me. They lurked just outside the corner of my eye; if I glanced their way, they also would run away, as if they didn't like being seen. (Of course, maybe they were just getting old and cranky, like the rest of us when we reach a certain age.) A few times I found myself addressing one of them, momentarily forgetting that I was asking for an opinion from a pile of clothing or perhaps quarreling with something as vague as a wisp of memory.

It all left me increasingly confused: How can anyone interact with an apparition—any kind of apparition—knowing all the while that it is both real and not real?

What did my neurologist think about all this? The truth is, since he never seemed interested in any of my hesitant inquiries, I never got around to mentioning my hallucinations to him. But all the while some unavoidable questions waited for their answers. Was I losing my mind? Had I lost it already? Was I avoiding pressing for a professional opinion because I was afraid of the answer? No, wait. I have to stop thinking that way.

One day in November, not long after the final radiation treatment, I parked the car in my garage and came through the back door to find all three of my children gathered in the living room, looking as if they were waiting for a bus they couldn't catch. They seemed mighty nervous about it, too. I was puzzled.

"What are you guys doing here?" I asked. "Is today a holiday or something?"

No answer: a lot more fidgeting.

"What is this…an intervention?" I joked.

"We don't think you should drive any more," John, the oldest, announced.

There was a general intake of air followed by dead silence, as if everyone was ready to duck under the table. It was an intervention, then. Could they be serious? Come on! Having grown up in the American Midwest meant that driving was the same as breathing. My father, as well as various uncles and cousins, had started me behind the wheel as soon as I could see over it—as early as thirteen or fourteen years old.

"What if I don't agree?" I asked.

"Then we have to talk about it," John replied.

So that's how it's done; first an appeal to reason, and if that fails, then—what? But okay, fair is fair. Let's try reason.

"We've all been watching you the last few months—maybe longer," John went on. "And we think you're an accident waiting to happen. Not to put too fine a point on it, as you always say."

"How do you mean, 'watching'?"

"We mean watching. Not spying, just picking up on things and then pooling our opinions."

"Dad," Corry chimed in, "do you remember that time you and Mom went to pick up that new mattress and you backed up through an empty lot straight into a concrete wall? You—"

"You said you'd lost your concentration," Jane said, interrupting.

"I remember...Well, I *had* lost my concentration. That doesn't make me a danger to man and beast."

"Or remember the time you nearly mowed down that cyclist on Harbord?" added John.

"Come on. That's not fair. That was as much his fault as mine. It was pitch black and he didn't have a light on his bike."

"That's true," Corry said. "But he also wasn't on the wrong side of the road."

John added, "And what about that little incident when you missed the 403 turnoff near Ancaster and pulled onto the wrong side of the freeway entrance? Do you happen to remember that?"

"Yeah, I remember. Shit, I thought you were going to reason with me."

"We haven't even come to that yet."

"Well, why don't you?" I snapped.

Silence.

Much as I wanted to deny it, I had to admit there was a lot of truth in their words. Not only that, there were several other incidents they didn't know about. I probably was going to maim someone if I kept driving. I flattered myself I would have eventually come to the same conclusion as the kids and done the right thing, but...I don't know. I could see it was obvious to everyone but me that something was wrong and that I couldn't keep endangering everyone else on the pavement. (I later found out that Corry was so concerned that she had written to the neurologist pleading for a diagnosis, asking him to at least give them a sense of how he was approaching my problems. She never received a reply.)

"Alright, alright," I finally conceded.

They had "won." But, I insisted that, if I were going to stop driving for the good of mankind, I would do it all at once. What the hell, I had given up smoking overnight forty-five years ago and never touched a cigarette since; I could give up driving the same way.

News flash: Quitting the road, it turns out, is harder than quitting cigarettes. Take my word for it. Smoking is merely an addiction; driving is how you get around, how you remain independent.

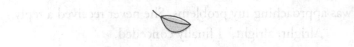

CHAPTER 4

Julie

Ken had mentioned the hallucinations when he first came home from the hospital after the TURP surgery. And there were his questions about "floaters" and "other people" in the room. I had plenty of questions of my own, but I'd been reluctant to quiz him when he was recovering from the TURP and then undergoing eight weeks of radiation treatment. One disease at a time, I told myself. But now, with the cancer worries finally out of the way, we were free to concentrate on the neurological side of things.

One languorous Indian summer day, not long after the move, we sat on the front porch contemplating the changing colors of the huge oaks, maples, and chestnuts that line our street. Out of the blue, Ken started to open up to me.

"It's getting bad lately. Maybe it's this place. It's so damn full of hallucinations—shapes turning into other shapes. You know...something like that," Ken revealed.

I said that maybe I could see what he meant. "Like when you're driving and you look at a faraway fence post that's covered with snow and for a moment you think it's a person standing there—something sort of like that?" I offered.

"No."

A pause. I tried again. "Okay, so what do you mean, then? Please talk to me. You have to tell me more if you want me to understand. When? Where?"

"It happens a lot. Especially when I get up at night."

"So what then? What happens? What do they do?" I persisted.

"They're just *there*," Ken said. "They come for me, until I chase them away."

As we talked, he seemed to visibly relax. By the time I stood up and went inside to make lunch, though, I thought this stuff must have been on his mind for a while. No wonder he had seemed so distracted lately. Though I had known about the apparitions, I hadn't realized how bothered he was by them.

Despite these troubling thoughts and my low stamina, I managed to get through the rest of the day's chores. Usually I am an excellent sleeper, but with Ken wandering the apartment at four a.m. (the same hour he disappeared the night after the operation), I was falling behind on my rest—seriously behind. Yogic breathing, counting backwards from a hundred, progressive muscle relaxation—none of the usual sleep techniques were working. My thoughts just refused to turn off.

Even after we began leaving a light on in the hall, Ken had trouble finding the washroom located right next to our bedroom. Once I woke to find him standing silently beside my side of the bed.

"I can't find the door."

I pointed to the open doorway, a bright yellow rectangle against the dark of the room, and he headed off. Another night, the plaintive inquiry, "What house are we in, anyway? It seems like I'm in two different houses."

After episodes like these, I would lie awake for hours as my mind posed and re-posed half-formed, unanswerable questions.

One afternoon, he expanded a bit more on the night visitors: "Sometimes I go up to them and poke at them, or even speak to them, and they just take off." I tried to picture myself in the same situation. As a child, I used to be frightened to go upstairs at night after listening to scary radio shows like "Lights Out" or "Inner Sanctum." At those times, my dad used humor to deflate my fears, telling me to be sure to check under the bed for monsters before I went to sleep. That tactic usually worked, but if there was a way of joking our way out of the present situation, I hadn't yet hit on it. "If I ever got up at night and encountered what you describe," I told Ken truthfully, "I'd run back to bed and pull the covers over my head like a three-year-old."

"But I'm a guy," he said and laughed. "I'm too brave for that kind of stuff."

In my search for enlightenment about Ken's symptoms, the obvious possibility of phoning the local Parkinson's Society hotline eventually occurred to me. The woman who answered the phone didn't sound surprised when I told her my story. "We're hearing more than we used to lately about the sort of thing you're describing," she told me. "The truth is that people are just beginning to pay attention to the cognitive issues that sometimes go with Parkinson's. Tell you what, if you'd like, I'll send you some literature."

A few days later, the postman pushed a bulky envelope through the mail slot. When I opened it, a wad of informational brochures and newsletters about every aspect of PD slid out. One sentence in "Taking Charge: A Guide to Living with Parkinson's," published by the Vancouver Coastal Health Authority, jumped out at me: "There are other conditions that share features of Parkinson's, and people living with these conditions may also find this information useful."

I reread that line several times before walking with brochure in hand to the computer. Three other conditions related to Parkinson's were listed. I Googled the first one, Multiple System Atrophy, scanned the description, and found the disease bore little resemblance to Ken's symptoms. Progressive Supranuclear Palsy, the second condition, was an even less likely candidate. (And given the scary-sounding nature of these two names, that was fine with me.) But when I typed in the odd-sounding "Lewy Body Dementia" (LBD), the results stopped me cold. It was described as a progressive disease, the three main features of which were: recurrent visual hallucinations, typically well formed and detailed; fluctuating cognition, with pronounced variable states of attention and alertness; and Parkinsonism.

Bingo! Triple bingo! A perfect fit! I couldn't wait to tell

Ken about my discovery; he had also been bothered by the lack of diagnosis. By the time he returned from his walk, however, I had thought better of telling him. If my layperson's diagnosis was wrong, I might upset him needlessly; if I was right, it was probably better that the news come from a healthcare professional.

In October, a third trip to the reluctant neurologist, a full year after the first, evoked a repeat of his maddening watch-and-wait approach. Fortunately, when we saw our family doctor, he listened patiently to our complaints and began talking about trying another specialist.

"I have someone in mind," Dr. Nguyen told us. "This guy is very smart, very articulate. You'll like him, I'm sure."

That was promising.

"And," he added with a reassuring smile, "he's having good results with some new medication."

I didn't need to hear more. How soon could we see the new man? Tomorrow? Over the next couple of weeks of waiting for a consultation, I was afraid to hope; we had lived so long in limbo between our first vague sense of something amiss and an actual diagnosis.

CHAPTER 5

Ken

In December 2007, I met the new doctor. He didn't refer to himself as anything like a neurologist: he called himself a psychiatric geriatrician. And I liked this soft-spoken, self-contained New Zealander. He actually listened when I spoke; he even appeared sympathetic when I enumerated my various symptoms, which ranged from mild tremor to half-crazy hallucinations.

The doctor made rapid notes as I let it all spill out, then reached into his desk and pulled out a book at which he kept glancing.

"What time of day do your hallucinations occur?" he asked. "How long do they last? What kinds of creatures appear in them? Where do the creatures go when they disappear? Do they speak to you or make any sounds at all? Are you having cognitive difficulties?"

At least I could say "no" to the last question. But I was dumbfounded; he, or at least his journal, possessed an uncanny ability to describe what had been racing through my half-cocked brain over the last few months. The symptoms he listed, right down to the smallest (imaginary) fluffy puppy scampering around our new apartment, seemed to have been copied directly from a hidden compartment of my cerebellum (hippocampus?). But if these manifestations were figments of somebody's overworked imagination (mine, presumably), how did they get into both of our brains? And how did this doctor know what I was going to say before I said it? How could he see into my head so clearly?

Now I'm too much of a rationalist to put my faith in imaginary figments, so I was pretty sure there had to be another answer. But sitting there in the doctor's office, in those first moments before I got hold of myself, I admit to being well and truly shaken. What baffled me most was that, judging by his notebook, other people were having *my* hallucinations.

Julie, whom the doctor called in for the last fifteen minutes of the hour-long consultation, had more than a few other details to add. Listening to her, I realized I had very little idea of what I had been putting my family through in the last several years.

But here is a new doctor, with a diagnosis in his back pocket. No hedging, no waiting for six more months. Sure as shootin' he knows what's wrong with me.

"You have Lewy Body Dementia with Parkinsonism," he announced in his quiet manner. *Lewy Body Dementia—of course! Now, why hadn't I thought of that?* Maybe because I'd never heard of it. Not that I had heard of Parkinsonism either, though I figured it must have some relation to Parkinson's disease.

Now, humor has always played a crucial role in my life. And although I don't find life quite as amusing I used to, I still prefer a doctor with a good sense of humor. I have developed a test to rate any new MD. So I tried it out on this man. Had he ever seen the Callahan cartoon where a nurse stands in the doorway of the doctor's waiting room facing one of the patients and announces, "The doctor will kill you now."

The geriatric psychiatrist laughed uproariously at the joke. Which, of course, led me to wonder what he knew that I didn't. What else was he hiding from me?

Julie

I'd been staring at the magazine for several minutes without any words registering when I heard a politely modulated voice ask, "Would you like to join us now?" I looked up to find the geriatric psychiatrist standing there. Once I was settled in a chair beside Ken, the doctor confirmed my Lewy Body suspicions and provided his own capsule summary of the disease for me.

"Do either you or Ken have any questions?" he asked. After giving brief to-the-point answers to our hesitant queries—the subject was still too new for us to be able to formulate anything much on the spot—he scribbled out a prescription form.

"I'm going to try you on Reminyl," he said to Ken. "It should help reduce some of your symptoms."

As we were putting on our coats, he ran his eye over his agenda and asked if we could come back in six weeks. *Six weeks instead of six months?* Yes, we could manage that. We left the office knowing that we still faced an uncertain future, but we were elated to finally have a name to put to Ken's strange assortment of symptoms.

Some among our acquaintance reacted with surprise when they heard the word "dementia." One nurse who had known us for years expressed dismay: "No! Not Mr. Sobol! It can't be!" A former classmate who lived in another city protested, "But Ken's as sharp as ever. Just the other day on the phone, he corrected me on the details of a story I was reminiscing about. He came up with names I'd totally forgotten!" Sometimes I just got a disbelieving look. As I struggled to come to grips with the daily reality of the new diagnosis, I found it hard to understand these people's apparent dismissiveness. (Much later, I realized that the very mention of the word "dementia" makes a lot of us uncomfortable.)

Luckily, I didn't lack emotional support on the home front. Old friends rallied round; our kids, now that we had a diagnosis (such a relief compared to that day back in June when we were just beginning to look for answers), came through wonderfully. John, who lives in Ottawa and wasn't able to travel to Toronto often told me, "Phone any time you need to talk, Mom, even at my work. Please, do not hesitate." I didn't hesitate, and he always made time. His wife, Annie, sent us long-distance vibes from Ottawa and provided an unfailingly upbeat note on family visits.

Corry got busy on the Internet. Over the next months she would prove invaluable at ferreting out helpful resources within the Toronto area. At this point in time, she was a stay-at-home mom with two teenagers, and though she got more than her fair share of requests for help, she performed them uncomplainingly. Corry's husband, Greg, not only phoned Ken with tickets to plays and Raptors games but also insisted on providing door-to-door chauffeur service.

Jane had a demanding job and a toddler with major health issues, yet she still displayed a helpful knack for providing *le mot juste* in any discussion. William, her husband, graciously rescued us from numerous household emergencies and from any computer problems that were beyond my scope.

But LBD's complex nature meant that even with close friends my replies to polite queries about Ken's health too often degenerated into vague mumblings. The symptoms had a conjurer's trick of showing up one day, hanging around awhile, and then suddenly *(Presto chango!)* disappearing. How to describe a day spent trying to come to terms with a disease whose overriding characteristic is inconsistency?

There was a limit to how much of this I wanted to dump on others, anyway.

Given such changed circumstances, our family and friends had their own relationships with Ken to work out. The younger generation, especially, already had a lot to handle; I had not forgotten the days when Ken and I tried to balance children, housework, cooking, careers, friends, and all the rest.

One day, while Ken was out on an errand, I went back to one of the websites I had found earlier, the one run by the Lewy Body Dementia Association, and began reading through a brief history of the disease. In 1912, the young German scientist Dr. Friedrich Lewy noted abnormal lumps of protein in a patient's brain. In 1919, another researcher, noting the same kind of clumps in a brain sample, named the phenomenon "Lewy Bodies" in honor of the man who first noted them. But it wasn't until 1996 that an international consortium proposed Dementia with Lewy Bodies as a distinct disease.

The overwhelming factor in LBD's physiology—as in some other similar degenerative neurological conditions—has to do with abnormalities in the brain's handling of proteins. What causes that mishandling in the first place wasn't clear to me from my quick survey, but a list of symptoms that followed was more to the point.

Like Alzheimer's, the article explained, LBD is progressive, incurable, and leads to progressive memory loss. Unlike Alzheimer's, however, LBD causes people to experience recurrent hallucinations, fluctuating cognition, and the motor

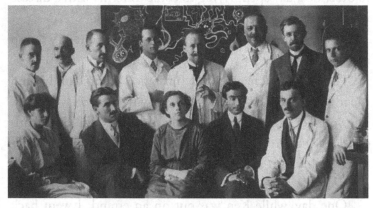

Munich, c. 1909: The scientists at this pathology lab include two key pioneers in dementia research: Dr. Alois Alzheimer (back row, third from right) who identified the first published case of "presenile dementia," later known as Alzheimer's Disease; and Dr. Friedrich Lewy (front row, far right), who first described the abnormal clumps he found in the brains of dementia patients. A later researcher would name these clumps "Lewy bodies" in honor of his predecessor.

symptoms of Parkinsonism (tremor and gait problems). Other symptoms of LBD include disorientation as to time and place, abnormal depth perception, emotional instability, fatigue, muscle stiffness, shuffling gait, daytime sleepiness, urinary difficulties, micrographia (small handwriting), hypomimia (blank face), and hypophonia (weak voice). As I read through the long list, I selfishly reminded myself that dementia is not a normal part of ageing, and that most people will never develop the disease.

On the same website, I found the magic words: "Caregivers' Forum." One click and up popped a treasure trove of helpful entries:

> Words are meaningless to someone who hasn't seen one of these LBD sufferers in action.... Visitors seldom come. [I] catch myself at times wondering if I'm being overly dramatic...friends announce, "Oh, he is doing so GREAT!" I feel not believed, isolated, and angry.

And this:
> Don is so much better when people are around that I feel that nobody else knows what my reality is...I tell them what's happening and they come for a visit expecting to find things going badly. Instead, Don responds to them by being very "on"...When I'm asked in front of him what's wrong...I can't really say, "Well he may look good now, but you should have seen him an hour ago." (Saying it behind his back would feel like a kind of betrayal.)

And another:
It felt so good to have my daughter tell me this summer…after spending 2 hours with Jack alone…that I had a toddler on my hands! She saw very little difference between the amount of energy required looking after her 18-month-old and Jack.

One website regular mused:
How is it that he can pick a piece of lint from my clothes but not see that the toilet needs flushing? That he can clear away the dish that I am still using, but not push in his chair? Where is the sense of it? The caregiver of a spouse with dementia must give up all rights to reason in the relationship. There is no room for reasonable. There is only "this is the way it is and will be."

Reading through these anguished cyber cries, I relaxed. I don't like tranquilizers and I'm not religious, so I can't turn to the bible when I'm feeling overwhelmed; but this fund of wise "web sisters" (men figured less often in the discussions) seemed to understand what I was going through. Over the next months, I would find myself revisiting the forum almost daily not only for answers but also for simple affirmations of my own reality. Had I lived in an earlier era, I wouldn't have had this kind of support.

I could just dimly recall my mother's description of family reunions in Lansing, Michigan, where her grandmother was kept busy scurrying around to answer the non-stop peevish demands of her wheelchair-bound husband.

And wasn't there something about him in one of those old letters? The recollection sent me rummaging through my store of family memorabilia until I found what I was looking for: a letter from my great-grandmother to my grandmother, the one after whom I was named.

Lansing, Michigan, June 7 [c. 1900]
Dear Julia,
I received your card today. I can't say anything very good of Pa; last night he was very anxious to go to bed early. In fact, he didn't sleep any to speak of all day although he was put on the couch and taken off nearly twenty times. Just loses himself and thinks he had lain down the greater part of the day. By the middle of the night, he was hallucinating, calling first one then someone else. And this forenoon it has been just the same. He don't seem to have any mind at all: I can't sit in the room with him without having to get up and do something for him every five minutes. I think our friends don't like to come here for all he does is ask them what they would do if they were just like he is, and don't they think he will be better pretty soon.

If Pa was quiet like Uncle Ed and slept a while during the day, why then it would not be so bad, for I could sew some besides doing the housework. I feel very much discouraged. I am not able to do very much and the way I live is very wearing. I wish very much I could see you all but I am afraid it would not be a good place for [you].

Love to all from mother.

As I read my great-grandmother's words, I was forcibly struck by how much the symptoms she mentioned—hallucinations, confusion, mobility issues, neediness—sounded like either LBD or perhaps a very advanced case of Parkinson's. And by now I had picked up enough family history to know that of her three daughters, one (Mary) had died early of appendicitis, another (Emily) had run off with a charming but questionable Irishman, and the third (Julia) had married and was living on a farm a half-day's journey from Lansing by train and buggy.

And today, here I sat at my computer, blessed to have my own daughters living just blocks away, my son instantly reachable by phone and email, access to free medical treatment from a whole array of physicians, and a new medication that if it didn't cure, at least promised to reduce Ken's symptoms. I was also scheduled to begin having a weekly housecleaning service subsidized by a local social agency, and that was not to mention the under-appreciated glories of electric light, hot showers, a washer and dryer, and the medical cornucopia of the worldwide web at my fingertips—none of which my great-grandmother could ever have imagined.

I feel a link with this isolated, hard-pressed, long-dead woman. I picture the time-travel scene: arriving one afternoon at the farmhouse, introducing myself to my bewildered great-grandmother, instructing her to put her feet up while I get the kettle on. While she naps in her chair after our conversation, I rummage around in the farm kitchen for the makings of the evening meal, maybe just an omelet and some fresh vegetables from her garden. After our supper, I stop by the couch and give my troubled great-grandfather a hug, then take my leave.

Fine talk. The truth is that in real time, as I deal with my own husband's troubles face to face, my patience is often failing me.

CHAPTER 6

Ken

All right, I give up. What exactly is a Lewy Body? How did I get LBD? How serious is it? And finally, the payoff—*What do I do about it?* I'll answer these questions as best I can, in reverse order based on what I've learned so far. But first, I should remind you that since people with dementia tend to mix things up, it's a matter of *sauve qui peut* in any conversation with me; form your own conclusions.

First question: What do I do about LBD? Not much, the doctors tell me. My disease will come and get me when it's ready, which could be as soon as three or four years from now, judging by the literature. If I'm very lucky, I could live considerably longer. Doctors have no way of predicting how serious my case is. There isn't a blood test, urinalysis, needle, or special x-ray machine that can deliver a definitive verdict.

The word on the ward is that usually four years pass between the point when symptoms are first noticed and actual diagnosis. My new doctor tells me he is pretty sure I'm in the early stage of LBD, but the rest is guesswork.

Who knows, I tell myself, maybe someone will come up with—not a cure, that's probably too far off to benefit me—but a treatment that can push the waiting period farther back and allow me to die of something else. The medication he has put me on, a relatively new drug called Reminyl (also known as galamantine), was originally intended to improve the quality of life for Alzheimer's sufferers. As things worked out, the drug more or less failed in that goal, but through anecdotal reports it was discovered to work brilliantly in the treatment of LBD. That's okay by me; it gives me hope that some scientist will make a new inadvertent but wonderfully helpful discovery that will help my case even more.

Next question: How serious is LBD? Pretty much comparable to Parkinson's, Alzheimer's, and the other incurable late-life brain diseases, except for the fact that it takes less time to kill you. Of course, it's possible the new drugs will extend life expectancy; but medications such as Reminyl are so recently developed that no one can claim to have an accurate read on them.

Third question: How did I contract my condition? As usual, there are lots of theories, but no one has a clear answer as to what triggers the symptoms. Though, here I have to admit that I misled you a bit earlier: there *is* one foolproof means of *identifying* the disease. Unfortunately, it involves two major drawbacks. First, the diagnosis can only be made during an autopsy; second, you are personally required to provide the cadaver. Unless you're willing to die for the cause, say good-bye to those dreams of starring in a renowned academic study that comes to the rescue. For now, all the medicos can do is watch you closely, mark down new symptoms as they appear, and put together a picture from the outside. It's screwball-comedy reasoning: people who get the disease get it because they're the kind of people who get it. Get it? Got it? Good. But that doesn't move medical science very far along.

Final question: What is a Lewy Body? That's a snap. A Lewy Body is "an abnormal deposit of a protein called alpha-synuclein in the part of the brain that controls thinking and movement." Put *that* in your corncob and smoke it.

Not long after our meeting with the new doctor, I was pleased to discover, from a newsletter Julie downloaded, that there are non-pharmaceutical techniques for keeping at least some symptoms at arm's length. One of the most annoying Parkinsonian aspects of the disease is the tendency for the vocal chords to shut down, sometimes so much so that speech becomes impossible. If you know me personally, you might recall I have a distinctive voice, at least to the extent that it generally gets recognized over the phone. No longer. Now I find myself having to insist on my identity while my oldest and dearest friends strenuously deny this could actually be me they are talking to. My voice has recently turned soft and sibilant, almost a whisper. If only I could remember to take that into consideration before the caller and I begin another belabored "Is that you? You sound different" dance of diseased syllables. For the most part, I barely remember to try.

Fortunately, singing helps strengthen the throat muscles,

and some farsighted people in Toronto have thought to organize a choir that any patient, caregiver, or person otherwise
associated with Parkinson's is warmly invited to attend. Julie,
Corry, and I decided to check out a choir rehearsal. I'm told
everyone is welcome, even if—like me—they've never sung
in a choir before. Julie has spent her life performing in highly
ranked choirs and Corry is a professional musician, but it has
always been assumed that the family musical talent reached
an abrupt cessation just before I opened my mouth.

You may wonder why I didn't join the local chapter of the
LBD Choral Society; the reason is that none exists. Though
experts insist LBD is the second-most common age-related
dementia after Alzheimer's (U.S. statistics say five million
people have Alzheimer's, one million people have LBD, and
eight hundred thousand people have Parkinson's), the disease
is little known even within the medical community. That's
because it was only recognized as a separate disease in the mid
1990s. In contrast, Parkinson's was isolated and described as
far back as 1817 and Alzheimer's around 1911. If you look
up those two conditions on your local library's website, you'll
find more self-help books and scientific studies than you
could ever get round to reading. The small number of pub-
lications on LBD, however, barely deserves its own category.

In February 2008, at the very first choir practice, I became
aware of a powerful and altogether beautiful male voice ema-
nating from behind me. *Whoa, Nellie! What had I got myself
into?* The voice turned out to belong to a retired physician
named Gordon Hardacre; and Gordon's wife, Enid, who sat
next to Julie, had equally impressive vocal talents.

While Julie took their talents in stride, I felt very much

like the neophyte chorister I was. I only relaxed a bit once we told Gordon and Enid that Julie and I had jointly written a history of the Lake Erie region. Since Gordon and Enid's son lives near the lake, they found the subject of special interest. In fact, when Gordon went home that night and Googled us he—being slightly naïve about this kind of stuff—mistook us for major writers. Who was I to disabuse him? Besides, that book had done quite well.

Gordon, I learned, had been forced by Parkinson's to put away his doctor's bag at the early age of fifty-eight. From what I've seen of him so far, he must have been a dynamite family doctor, one of those well-loved types you sometimes come across in the obits and wonder how on earth did he or she have time for all those accomplishments when I can barely manage to peel the carrots for dinner. But his illness had put paid to most of his activities. On bad days, Gordon's palsy is so pronounced you practically have to nail him down to hold a conversation.

Gordon and I talked about driving during a break one afternoon not long after I had joined the choir. He confided that he, too, had pretty much given it up, though the other day he caved in to his automotive urges (which sounded quite similar to mine). He'd wheeled the car out of the garage and spent the entire afternoon blasting up and down the freeways of southwestern Ontario. I'm sure he was exaggerating, but the very thought of being on the same road with another rip-roaring, not-completely-in-control driver like myself scared me half to death.

I haven't driven since.

Julie

Chronic disease is an uninvited guest that moves into your home and then proceeds to act as if it's the host and you're the guest. "*I'll* set the rules," the intruder tells you, standing in front of the door with arms folded tightly. "And please to remember, there is no room for reasonable now. There is only 'this is the way it is.'"

Moreover, each person has to work out his or her own *modus vivende* for sharing the house with the intruder/disease. Reminyl had helped Ken by reducing the number of hallucinations, but the night creatures hadn't disappeared completely. Neither had the "variable cognition" phenomenon nor the executive function deficit.

When we first moved back to Toronto, Ken and I had begun work on a third book, one that required extensive research. The manuscript's complex structure involved frequent jumps in time and place, and as the months passed, and Ken's memory became shakier day by day, it became obvious that navigating our way through these challenges was impossible. We put the manuscript away, and then took it out a few days later for another try before reluctantly shelving it for good. This was a major loss, piled on top of others.

Fortunately, staring us in the face was what seemed to both of us a more manageable subject, one that would involve no travel and little research: the ongoing story of a personal encounter with a disease no one we knew had ever dealt with—or, for that matter, ever heard of.

We got to work quickly, and this time the process went better.

But so much change, so much change. Take, for example, the car. I have been driving since I was sixteen, and have logged countless hours of driving on country roads over the last few years. But Toronto streets are an obstacle course: new bike lanes, speed bumps, pedestrian crossings, plus the sudden screeching halt of streetcars and disgorging of passengers in the middle of the road mean you always have to be on the alert. Now I was coping with the additional challenge of a nervous backseat driver.

Our kids' confrontation with Ken had the desired effect of keeping him from behind the wheel; I was glad of that. But though they had left with smiles on their faces that evening, I knew he wasn't as sanguine as he appeared. He was good at covering up his symptoms in front of other people—even our children—but I knew his anxiety level about all these changes in his life was rising.

"What are you doing!" he shouted as I brought the car to a stop during one post-intervention outing. "Don't ever pull up right next to a bunch of policemen!!"

The uniformed trio in question, bicycles at their sides, were standing next to a bright-red Stop sign to which Ken was completely oblivious. I could picture the scene if I had followed his suggestion: me speeding past the group, followed by a high-speed chase through the neighborhood, cyclists and pedestrians racing to get out of the way. Tomorrow's accusatory newspaper headlines would read: "Grandmother Nearly Mows Down Mother With Stroller," "Get Senior Drivers Off Our City Streets," and "Speed Kills: Do Seniors Need Yearly Driving Tests?"

Ken fretted that I was driving too fast, too slow. We

would be late, we would be early. We were going down the wrong street, or headed in the wrong direction. Trips to the supermarket became increasingly testy. Finally, as we returned home one day through heavy traffic, the backseat crammed with grocery bags, I told Ken it might be best if he stayed home next time.

"People can't concentrate if they're not left in peace to use their own judgment," I explained. "It's really a question of basic road safety, nothing personal."

He nodded glumly. We had been enjoying these weekly excursions. Even a meander through the overstocked aisles of a stadium-sized supermarket can look good when you're housebound much of the time.

The new regime didn't last long, but when we resumed our joint outings, I found the break had helped. "A small victory," I wrote to my old college friend, Jane, in New York. "The secret is mental preparation and lots of deep breathing once you're out on the road," I added.

"Small, but not so small, really!" Jane wrote back.

Ken was still uncomfortable in the passenger seat, and each time the garage door creaked shut behind us, he was convinced its metal edge would chop the car in half (and maybe take our heads with it). But he worked at keeping his fears under control. As I pulled into our spot one day, he surprised me by asking, "How do you do that—gauge when to turn the wheel? I could never get that right!" That was a good moment.

And Jane was right: victories of any size deserve to be celebrated. You need to keep them handy for the bad moments. These days, I often found myself giving way to tears in unpredictable places—cafes, children's school performances, and even (most embarrassingly) while stretched out in the dentist's chair as she calmly outlined the pros and cons of a complex procedure that might include two root canals, gum surgery, and a crown (all to save one tiny tooth).

How do I unravel the threads? How do I tease out the underlying cause of an emotion? How many of these salty drops were for Ken, I wondered, and how many for myself? How many for the ever-evolving list of daily duties as, week by week, my husband loses the ability to manage the most basic tasks? How many for what all this change will mean for our children and grandchildren? How many for the never-to-be-regained hours of sleep, for the lost spur-of-the-moments outings, for just being able to jump in the car and drive?

All this self-questioning dredges up a long-forgotten school-yard incident.... *"What are you crying for, little girl?"*

I look up to find the school principal, Mr Heavenridge (his real name) looming over me. We are standing on the wide walkway in front of the school, surrounded by kids shouting and jostling. It takes me a while to stop sniffling long enough to answer his question.

"I've lost my hat. It—it—hurts."

"What hurts?"

"My ear. My ear hurts."

Earache, for any reader lucky enough never to have experienced that sensation, is a peculiarly intense pain, sharper and deeper even than the one caused by the dental drill in those spare-the-novocaine days. And my mother had often lectured me on the folly of going hatless in a cold wind. "That's a good way to get an earache, Julie. Or if you already have one, it's a good way to make it worse," she would say.

*Mr. H. studies me for a moment, considers, leans down.
"Take off your jacket for a minute, Julie."
I obey without questioning and stand there shivering and wondering what's next. Kids stop their ball-tossing and rope-skipping and gather to watch as, like a magician triumphantly pulling a rabbit from a top hat, he reaches inside the sleeve, extracts the knitted wool cap from where I must have put it, ties the strings neatly under my chin. All chivalry, he helps me into my jacket, then winks at me before heading back inside to face whatever it is that principals do, and everyone goes back to their games.*

I don't recall whether those few hatless moments led to another bout of ear poking and lancing and head-shaking from the doctor, or to the prescribing of more pills. I'd like to think not. I prefer to think that this simple act of kindness by a busy adult saved me from a repeat of that pattern of pain and evil-tasting medicine. With the fight against the Nazi war machine at its height, men and women were pouring into the Detroit area to take their place on assembly lines turning out bombers and tanks in the huge River Rouge and Willow Run plants. In my school, with teachers facing classes of forty or more, classrooms were so crowded that some kids had to sit in the hall. On days when the weather made recess an impossibility, the place was bedlam. Mr. H. had more on his mind than lost hats.

I'm an adult now, and if someone asked me, "What are you crying for, dear?" the answer would be harder to come by. Like anyone forced to deal with unpredictable, overwhelming change, I wanted my/our life back, the life we had lived, debated, planned, and nurtured for more than forty years. But it didn't look as if anyone—not even Ken's sympathetic geriatrician, the closest thing we had to a Mr. Heavenridge—was going to pull any rabbit out of any hat, or any hat out of any sleeve. Today's term is "anticipatory grief." My tears are for present pain and the pain to come.

I vented to anyone who could stand to listen. When people said, "You have to get out more," I obediently grabbed my jacket and headed out. Our neighborhood is a wonderful place for walking because of the varied architecture and people you pass on the sidewalks—seniors like us, young parents pushing complicated strollers, university students, business people, new immigrants, and late in the afternoon clots of high school kids chatting and jostling their way home. Every day the mix is different.

I also made a point of inviting new acquaintances for lunch; if one of them recommended a book, I got hold of a copy and sat down and read it. Web blogs are fine as far as they go, but for a deeper look there's nothing like a book.

When I read *To Love What Is*, Alix Kates Shulman's account of how she and her husband coped after he sustained major brain damage in an accident, I couldn't put it down. Although the onset of Alix's husband's condition had been sudden rather than gradual, the problems they faced, from work challenges to tussles with medical staff to the rearrangement of the furniture in their small apartment, were not so different from the ones we were dealing with. I finished the book in one sitting.

One of the articles in a Parkinson's Society newsletter helped, too. Dr. Gordon Hardacre, a soon-to-be friend, wrote about a newly formed choir, directed by a retired minister whose mother had suffered from Parkinson's. The group was looking for members.

We were also looking, looking for more structure to our increasingly disordered lives, and weekly choir practices sounded like just the ticket.

Ken had never done any kind of group singing, unless you counted his participation in impromptu singsongs led by various Clancy Brothers back in the days when we hung out in Greenwich Village and the beer was flowing freely in the White Horse Tavern on a Saturday night. But he was willing to give it a try. Corry, when she heard of our plans, volunteered to sing, too, and act as our designated driver. Good. One less thing to think about.

I wasn't sure what to expect when we entered St. Timothy's Church Hall for the first time. A single row of chairs stretched across the width of the large, high-ceilinged room; metal walkers stood next to a couple of seats. A few people sat quietly, sorting through their music, while others stood around in clusters talking animatedly. I couldn't tell who among the crowd might be a Parkinson's patient and who a friend or family member.

After spotting us, a smiling woman detached herself from one of the clusters and hurried over. "Hello. I'm Bruna, and

you must be the Sobols. We've been expecting you." Others
started wandering over to be introduced, but just then the
director played a few notes on the piano, and we found ourselves in the middle of what looked like a game of musical
chairs as everyone scurried for a seat. As soon as the director
raised his arm, people sang

Doh
Doh, ti
Doh, ti, la,
*Doh, ti, la, sol…*and so on, down the diatonic scale.

I was knocked over by the intensity of the sound. The
room had good acoustics, but it was more than that; there was
a real joy in the music, even in this simple warm-up exercise.

The group launched into the first song, with Paul Walker,
the director, doubling as accompanist. I was transfixed as
cascades of atonal chords, chords that could have been
written by Mahler or Stravinsky, poured out of the grand
piano. Amazingly, these harmonies blended with the bouncy
Newfoundland sea chantey everyone was practicing. Evidence
that real musicianship was at work here.

On the way home, as Corry navigated the car through
the afternoon rush hour, she said, "Dad, I could hear you
clearly, and you actually have a very pleasant voice. You even
sang on key." Ken was both surprised and pleased. What I
found surprising, though, was that he agreed with me when
I remarked on what a congenial bunch they seemed. Usually
he shuns all forms of group activity. It probably helped that
he is a good sight-reader, but I think it was mostly a question of motivation (the choir needed him and he needed the

choir) and the fact that he loves music. Here was a chance to participate without feeling judged.

Over the next few weeks, Ken found the choir challenging in ways that had nothing to do with people or vocal ability. Every time the conductor announced a new song, Ken was left shuffling through his folder while the rest of the choir politely stood around, trying to look as if they had nothing better to do. Managing the slippery pile of sheet music was hard at best. Even Corry's attempt to rearrange his folder in alphabetical order, using colored tabs for each letter of the alphabet, didn't help. Nevertheless, he soldiered on. After repeated practices, he had the words by heart, and with the other members encouraging him and Gordon's ringing voice for inspiration, the paper chase became less of a worry. By the time the choir broke for the summer, the Sobols had participated in two well-received performances, and our fellow singers were beginning to seem very much like friends.

CHAPTER 7

Ken

It shouldn't come as a surprise to hear that dementia patients become increasingly confused in their dealings with the outside world. I often get into situations where I am required to take an either metaphorical or literal number before joining a long queue. Not until my number is called do I realize that I've managed to lose my damn ticket somewhere between the beginning and end of what, on second viewing, is actually a short line. People quietly snarl and glare before I can finally locate my number in a back pocket—that is, if I ever manage to find it.

But people sometimes surprise me by proving unexpectedly civilized and helpful when I'm struggling. For example, there's the genial manager of my local newspaper store, a Syrian man whom I have known casually for years and who is never in a hurry as far as I can tell. I was at his front counter the other day when I drew a total blank about the name of the magazine I had come in to purchase. Miracle of miracles, it turned out he was reading an article on Parkinson's disease in an Arabic-language newspaper; he told me that he recognized in me some of the symptoms. When I confirmed he was right, or close enough, he ignored the half-dozen other customers; they stood patiently as he questioned me in detail about my problems, even drawing in some of the other customers. Of course, you can't count on this kind of serendipitous coincidence occurring more than once in a lifetime. You must always be prepared for your next public humiliation. Or just close your eyes and hope—it's as useful as anything else.

Let me show you what I mean. A few days ago, I needed something from the local hardware store. The elderly gent who served me behind the counter was a bit doddery (*I* should talk). When he tried to hand me change, the coins spilled out all over the counter and floor. "Shit," the man murmured as he lowered himself to the floor on a matched pair of arthritic hands and knees. As he located each coin, he would reach up and put it slowly into my hand; but at least half of them had rolled under the ancient display cases, never to be seen again. When he shook his head and looked as if he were about to cry, I knew exactly how he felt. The word humiliation doesn't express the half of it.

Eventually, his wife wandered out from the back. After taking in the situation, she leaned across the counter, opened the cash register, and reached inside for a new supply of change, all the while rolling her eyes at both me and her husband and grudgingly allowing that she would clean it all up later. The clerk started to protest, but soon gave up. It was just then that I noticed the pronounced tremor in his right hand. I felt terrible, as if I had been the author of this entire depressing episode. Picking up my purchase, I slipped out as quickly and quietly as I could.

In my own case, up till now, little had been happening on the palsy front. Then tremor-hell broke loose. The shaking in my hands became almost constant. And, if that weren't enough, I'm beginning to find that in social interactions, whether with an old acquaintance, a neighbor, or a store clerk, I've become a victim of another joker in the LBD deck. I never know how I will feel five minutes from now. What starts out as a cheerful, perhaps even thoughtful, morning can quick as a cat slide into a black dungeon of a noontime. My mood changes are not dramatic—like a crash of thunder—but they feel like it. They come on me suddenly as I stand admiring a newly planted bed of flowers or while at a street corner casually waiting for the light to change.

In the final pages of *Pride and Prejudice*, when Elizabeth Bennet teases Darcy by demanding to know precisely when and why he fell in love with her, Darcy can only say he doesn't know. He was, he freely admits, in the middle of things before he knew love had begun. That's not a bad description for how I feel about LBD's constantly changing moods: I can't find any rhyme or reason for any aspect of it.

Julie

It was now the summer of 2008. In the months since the diagnosis, Ken and I had learned something about LBD, and this small store of increased knowledge brought with it an increased ability to cope. I liked to picture our life as a graph: one jagged downward-sloping line charting the inevitable progression of this difficult disease and another line climbing upward to represent our hard-won (but reasonably steady) climb toward acceptance. On good days—of which we were experiencing many, despite my gloomy talk—I thought we were coping pretty darn well with our unwelcome visitor. On bad days (no shades of gray here, just good and bad)...well, we just got on with it.

At least with the long, icy winter well out of the way, we could take our worries outside. There were no open skies and wide fields dotted with woodlots to draw our gaze outward, but our street had plenty of trees leafing themselves back to life. Seated again on the front porch, reveling in the flower-scented air (the lilacs and forsythias in some of these front yards look as if they could date from the same era as the many-gabled houses), it seemed to me that even LBD's tight grip lightened just a little.

I was reading the newspaper outside one warm day when an item in the paper's advice column caught my attention. A reader explained that she was recovering from a devastating pancreatic illness. The poor woman had undergone twenty-six hospitalizations, and a pancreas transplant. She had nearly died in the process; her marriage broke up. Why was it, she wanted to know, that so many people downplayed her situation, as if she only had a bunion removed? It seemed a fair question. The columnist answered that many people don't even want to think about things like a dangerous surgery, either because they're squeamish, or they feel they're intruding if they ask too many questions, or because they just don't know how to deal with a friend's pain.

People who send a card are at least showing interest, she pointed out, even if not on the level you might like; and the ones who tell you to "snap out of it" probably think their words of encouragement are helpful. "Try," she wrote, "to worry less about them. Focus on yourself." I could almost feel the light going on in my brain. I thought of the young man we had worked with who had apologized profusely because he didn't go to visit Ken during his cancer treatments. "I just don't do well with hospitals," he explained shamefacedly, though no explanation was necessary.

Why should I have been so surprised by people's reactions (or lack of them) to Ken's LBD diagnosis? At least the word pancreas is dimly familiar from high school science classes. But even months after the diagnosis, *no one* we had run into, apart from patients and their health care providers, had ever heard of a Lewy Body. Adding to the confusion was the fact that a) Ken's only obvious physical symptom was a mild tremor, and b) dementia patients possess an uncanny knack for pulling themselves together when others are around (a phenomenon known as "show time" in the LBD online forum). No wonder friends, let alone casual acquaintances, often failed to pick up on the signals.

As for the hallucinations, which doctors consider the most telling symptom of LBD, I was finding that any mention of them in social situations caused an awkward silence unless some conversationally adept soul heaved the discussion on to another topic. Ken, however, once he got over his reluctance to talk about the hallucinations, began to take a certain delight in stopping the conversation dead by telling a guest, "I'm surprised you didn't notice that mouse (or ferret, or newt, or bat, or snake) crawling up your pant leg." Joking aside, these small animal sightings, which seemed to come out of nowhere and appeared in broad daylight, troubled Ken more than the fanciful night creatures.

Even a century after Freud's *Psychopathology of Everyday Life*, and despite Hollywood's occasional attempts to deal sympathetically with the subject, people are still uncomfortable around diseases involving the mind. Alzheimer's, which has a more straightforward trajectory, has gained considerable attention from filmmakers. Sarah Polley's *Away From Her* is one good example. But some neurological diseases aren't as easily summed up, or as easily glamourized. With such complex conditions as LBD, Pick's Disease, Huntington's, Frontal Lobe Dementia, Progressive Supranuclear Palsy, or Multiple System Atrophy, the story—and the audience—tend to get lost in the telling.

Sometimes life can be too painful, too subtle, and too complex to turn into a successful film script. Maybe some day.

Ken
Even the language surrounding LBD carries a heavy burden. Early on, a social worker had inquired whether I found the use of the term "dementia" too disturbing. *Too disturbing to do what?* I wondered. If the answer was "so disturbing that you want to flee from the Lewy Body Club," well, it was too late; my seat on the boat was already booked. But after giving the question more thought, I concluded that the answer is "yes."

Yes, I do find the term "dementia" too close to "demented" for comfort. And then "yes" again, because dementia would prove extremely difficult to de-stigmatize. But finally, "no. I don't." A neutral vocabulary is essential if we are to get anywhere in educating people about diseases such as Parkinson's, Alzheimer's and LBD. "Dementia" is all we've got at the moment.

It was a different social worker who eventually made me aware of another problem: Julie's growing need for respite. The social worker convinced me that, in my absorption with my own troubles, I had unthinkingly dumped the work of managing all the medical paperwork, keeping track of my varied medications, deciphering online instructions when the computer got balky, and all the other minutiae of modern life onto my wife. Julie doesn't have much stamina at best, and all it took was one long glance for me to see that, at seventy-two, she was aching with exhaustion. (I won't say she hadn't been complaining: she had been—loudly and vociferously. I simply had not been listening or looking.)

After the social worker left, Corry made some calls. Somebody who knew somebody who knew somebody else who knew how these things were arranged got to work, and a few days later I heard myself agreeing to spend one day a week at a nearby adult daycare center, a place for not-exactly-lost souls but not-precisely-"found" ones either.

When I first walked through the door at St. Christopher House in November 2008, I couldn't imagine what I was doing there. However, I reminded myself, at the very least I would be giving Julie a chance to put her feet up for a few hours. On the first day there, the staff was in the midst of organizing a go-round among the thirteen clients who had showed up. This was a Friday—always a slow day, I was told. The first thing item on the agenda was the suggestion that each of us in turn explain where we were born and how we arrived at where we are now.

One elderly man (I took him to be Polish) was so deep into the final stages of Alzheimer's that he was past coherency in any language. (He turned out to be from Portugal and was familiar to many in the group as a once well-known bandleader in Lisbon.) Another man, who had worked for years as the captain of a fishing boat, burst into tremulous, distressed (and distressing) tears when it was his turn to speak. He didn't know where he'd been born, despite the staff's encouragement. However, they seemed to be expecting his reaction: three or four workers rushed over to wrap him in hugs.

I tried drifting around in the wake of a middle-aged South Asian woman as she paced the floor muttering to herself in English about her origins, hoping to understand a sentence or two. Suddenly, she flounced out of the room. The remaining nine were all elderly Portuguese immigrants, none of whom spoke English well enough to carry on a conversation. They had all emigrated from the same small village on the same small island in the Azores—and all at around the same time, just in case that wasn't coincidence enough.

At that point, all I wanted to do was leave and be amongst my own people, whoever they were. I still had no answer as to how and why I had landed here. Who, exactly, had sent me? Even the people in charge had looked baffled when I showed up, though they had womanfully banded together to make me feel sort of welcome. (But no hugs…yet.) All of them, beginning with Jean Nogueira, the youthful and lively boss of the program, insisted on taking me on a tour of the three large connected rooms where the activities, ranging from field trip planning to bingo games to lunch preparation, were crammed.

The fact that you could get a clear view of any of these rooms from any position was strategic, I discovered later. The doors are kept locked (only staff members have keys) to prevent breakouts or clients from wandering away. To my surprise, this rule also applied to me, should I choose to sign on. I had thought I was special. You know, cultured and cool and all that. No one else seemed to have noticed.

Another reason I was left scratching my head that first day was everyone's insistence that I come back when Donald was there. Donald didn't come on Fridays, but he was the one to keep an eye out for. Donald was "the man." Donald would clear everything up. We were as similar as could be: two peas in a pod, Donald and me. I just shrugged and assumed that Donald must be some kind of social worker—a man hugger to balance out the women.

When I got to meet him on my second visit, I quickly realized my mistake. Donald wasn't one of "them" but one of "me." The workers were absolutely right. Donald is a hulking, two-hundred-and-thirty-pound cluster of sharp intelligence and The-Man-Who-Came-to-Dinner-type crabbiness. He has Parkinson's, diabetes, one leg, and no real teeth, in addition to being legally blind and deaf. Yet Donald manages to keep up his spirits far more bravely than I do mine. No wonder the staff wanted me to meet him. Everyone there—staff or client—wants him to stay around, at least until they bite the dust themselves. It's an honor to have him in your neighborhood drop-in center.

To be truthful, I expected to become one of those would-be escapees in double-quick time, but something unlikely happened. I found myself becoming fond of the people at St. Christopher House. Though few of them could speak English, and all I could do was count up to ten in their language, we somehow got along.

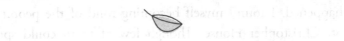

CHAPTER 8

Julie

One day I chanced upon a British website related to Ken's condition. (In England they put the word dementia first, as in Dementia with Lewy Bodies; but it's the same disease.) The site lacked an online forum, but made up for that by offering up a selection of informative short videos. Watching a television actress from the popular EastEnders series describe her husband's struggle with the disease moved me to tears, but it was another film that really grabbed my attention.

A white-coated lab worker holds up a slide with a piece of somebody's brain smeared onto it. The camera cuts to a close-up of what looks like a Miró painting, filled with blobs and swirls, or a photo of some past-the-expiry-date scrambled eggs, as researcher Dr. Ian McKeith describes how something as simple as an improved staining method led lab workers to view LBD as a distinct disease. The blobs are clumps of protein that form in an LBD patient's brain—not the good kind of protein extolled in "how to eat healthy" articles but something that definitely does not belong there. An ominous version of the "one of these things is not like the other" game you see on Sesame Street.

McKeith sums up LBD in one pithy sentence: "Dementia with Lewy Bodies is really very different from most dementias because it imposes multiple burdens for the patient to deal with, making it hard to plan even an hour ahead." He also tells us that relatives often rate the quality of life of the patient as worse than death.

Despite all this, the doctor sees cause for optimism. McKeith believes the disease will turn out to be one of the more treatable forms of dementia. "In Alzheimer's," he explains, "you get 'demented' because cells die, irreversibly die, and there's not much you can do about that. In DLB you probably get the dementia because cells aren't working properly, which is why it fluctuates. There's more potential to improve and treat." McKeith has begun collaborating lately with the scientist Walter Schulz-Schaeffer, who believes he is close to figuring out what causes the cells to stop working.

This little film is the first bit of hopeful news that anyone has given us, and, though he doesn't know it, the optmistic Dr. McKeith has become our friend for life. Given his hopefulness, it's not surprising that he always makes a point of telling caregivers about the website before they leave his clinic (I had to learn about it on my own). And incidentally, for anyone interested in the larger picture, the doctor describes one of the global implications of LBD. As life expectancy in developing countries increases day by day, he points out, "It really falls to us to find solutions before the world's population becomes enormous."

Back at the local level, though, Ken and I live mainly in the present. Our social life has taken on a neurological bent; among the people we hang out with these days is a former classmate whose father died after a long struggle with Parkinson's, a woman whose brother suffers from a fast-moving version of Parkinson's (he was confined to a wheelchair just months after his diagnosis), and a California artist whose family worked in the film business and whose father's colorful hallucinations include a set of song-and-dance men right out of the old musicals.

Then there is Gourete Broderick, a Toronto woman whose fellow volunteers in the Lewy Body Dementia Association have nicknamed "Mother Courage." In 2005, that organization (American-based but used by Canadians and people around the world) named Gourete their Volunteer of the Year. She received the award because she became so incensed about the disease's low profile that, while helping care for a mother with LBD, she undertook her own information campaign. Gourete emailed brochures on the subject to some four thousand medical professionals worldwide, printing and sending out a thousand brochures within the Toronto area alone, with plans to expand her work across Canada. I've met Gourete a couple of times and learned a lot about the disease just by talking to her.

Yes, I place high value on the work of researchers like Dr. McKeith as well as the other neurologists, geriatricians, psychiatrists, and so forth who do what they can for dementia patients. Without their intimate knowledge, both academic and personal, of the human body, and especially the brain, we would be at a loss. But once a diagnosis is made and a pill prescribed, patients and caregivers desperately need follow through. Volunteers who set up and run websites and organize fundraising marathons, family practitioners who help families interpret the specialists' medical jargon, social workers who provide a willing ear and practical advice when crises arise, physical therapists, speech therapists, day program workers, personal care workers—they all play a part in filling in the cracks left by the specialists. Just the fact that Silvana (housekeeper) and Nati (respite worker) show up on time for their weekly two-hour stints and are unfailingly courteous is worth a lot to me, but they also get the work done. Without them, my situation would be more like my great-grandmother's, an uncomfortable thought.

Not long after the diagnosis, Ken had commented, "It's very hard on you, I can see that now. Later, it will be harder on me." He's always been given to making dire pronouncements, but this one was right on. We've made it through another year with Mr. Lewy Body, but I watch with distress as the disease takes an ever-increasing toll on his daily functioning.

Ken was always the noisiest member of the family. ("Corry excepted," he would add.) Not anymore. "Use your BIG voice," the speech therapists like to say. That advice is helpful if you want—really want—to ask someone to pass the salt. But in a real conversation, such self-conscious effort puts constraint on off-the-cuff wit. These days Ken speaks less, often drifting away into a world of his own at social gatherings. As for his handwriting, never a model of penmanship, you would need a magnifying glass to make out a single word.

The tremor is increasing. I can hear the rattle-tattle-tattle of the newspaper from the next room, and though it's painful to hear, I know it's more painful to experience. In restaurants, it's hard for us to ignore the occasional rude stare or quickly redirected glance. By evening, his over-exercised wrists ache. The Levocarb prescribed by a new neurologist seemed to reduce the shaking at first, but nothing is simple with LBD. When the dosage was increased from two to three pills a day, Ken's waking dreams returned in full living color, and he went back to the lesser dose.

I used to like hearing my father sing around the house; he favored comic ballads picked up from the Hit Parade, sentimental Victorian plaints like "The Letter Edged in Black," folk songs about the whistle of a train coming down a long, impossibly lonesome track. (Train songs always seem to be lonely.) I miss the sound of his off-tune warble as he came down the stairs for supper. Sometimes my father sang for the joy of it, sometimes, so it seemed to my younger self, in defiance of personal demons. My early awareness of music's power to raise the spirits has been reinforced by our participation in a choir whose common thread is a shared interest in neurological illness. If a medication works, that's great; hooray for Reminyl! However, music *always* helps and carries neither cost nor side effect.

"I happened to mention that you played the piano," Ken told me one day after returning from his day program. "Now Jean wants you to come and play for group singing sessions."

A couple of weeks later, I sat down at St. Christopher's creaky but in-tune upright. Picking what looked like an easy piece, "Rosa d'Alexandria," from the songbook, I began playing. The response was immediate. This group needed no warm-up to launch into a set of Portuguese favorites—they all knew the songs by heart, and some were fine vocalists. I had no idea what they were singing about so rousingly as we moved on through "Nas Voltinhas de Marão," "Ó Ciranda," and such sweetly mournful tunes as "Vira Do Minho" (my personal favorite), but their muscular musicality transported me to the Azores for the afternoon.

At one point, Edwardia ventured a solo in a throaty Edith Piaf contralto. Gerveze, a former opera singer, executed a few intricate dance steps as he performed a few lines from an Italian aria. When somebody requested "You Are My Sunshine," everyone joined in, including the staff. And so it went. When Jean walked over to thank me as I got up to leave, I told her I had probably enjoyed the experience more than the singers. (I have had the same feeling on each of my subsequent visits.)

Humor is another weapon against self-pity. A few years back, we reconnected with a Canadian animator whom Ken had known at Filmation Studios during our three-year stay in California. Paul Crudden was a talented artist, but the heady days when they worked together on a series of shows, including one based on Julies Verne's *Journey to the Center of the Earth*, were long past. Since then, Paul had fought a losing battle with alcohol and had come on hard times.

At the facility where he was living after a stroke, we listened as he explained—a slow, painful process—that his social worker had given him a name of a speech therapist and suggested he call her. Paul was willing enough, he told us, but when the woman answered the phone she had so much trouble making sense of his wheezes, grunts, and other incomprehensible noises that she finally hung up.

"She probably thought I was drunk or a newcomer who didn't speak a word of English," Paul explained, breaking into laughter as he spoke. "But, anyway, I decided that if they couldn't manage to understand me at a speech clinic, my case was hopeless." We laughed with him as his thin body shook with guffaws.

We don't get out a lot these days, but we take our jokes where we can find them, which is mostly through the magic shadows of the small screen. Away from the television, we share our own private comedy channel. The oft-repeated What Have You Done With My Keys? routine that ends with Ken's Yogi Berra punchline, "But if I don't find them, I might lose them," gets a big laugh from its audience of two. Though maybe you have to be living the situation to truly grasp the subtlety of the humor.

A new year, 2009.
"When memories disappear, make new ones," the adage goes. Our family is doing its best. On Februrary 5th, a new grandchild presented herself to the world, and in the charmingly direct way of babies, began demanding her own place at gatherings. "I'm Lara, and I'm here! Pay attention!" she seems to say. We have also managed a few short excursions, mainly to the countryside. A midwinter day trip to our old haunts along Lake Erie, the shoreline a waste of ice. A week last August at

a cottage in the Kawarthas where eight adults, five children, and two dogs come, go, swim, eat, sleep, talk, and canoe in different permutations. A visit to a forested provincial park where we stood with daughters and granddaughters on the top of a large dam, a manmade lake behind us and the tumbling river emerging below on the other side, to gaze out over the million or so shades of green. A few weeks ago, Ken and I took a trip to Ottawa by train for a visit with John, Annie, and their two kids. In these different groups and settings, our family is getting to know each other in new and sometimes surprising ways.

I think I am doing better, in a sink-or-swim kind of way, at keeping awkward conversations going. The challenge is good for me, I tell myself, and admittedly I enjoy voicing my opinions more. Still, how I miss hearing Ken's forceful voice chiming in on whatever subject is at hand! I haven't always agreed with his opinions, but from our first date, I have consistently found them to be rooted in a deep moral sense and a keen appreciation of human psychology. I work at refraining, when asked how things are going, from launching into a summary of the week's ups and downs. *Keep it short*, I tell myself. *Answer the question behind the question*: "The medicine is helping, thanks for asking;" "Every day is different, but we're coping;" and "It's been a challenging week, but we have lots of good days. Really."

All true and not quite true at the same time.

Ken

I read a lot as a kid. Right from the start, it seemed to me that the four words, "Yo, I'm a writer," in answer to the query,

"And what do *you* do?" comprised the baddest exchange of banter the English language had to offer. I still feel that way.

At the age of twenty-one, I was fortunate enough to start publishing regularly in the *Village Voice* in New York. Few of my friends and colleagues have ever understood how much of a validation that was for me. The writing gig ultimately led to fifteen years of on-the-job training, years that taught me more than any "J-school" ever could. Then nearing the end of a reasonably successful career—let's say as early as 2002—something happened. Suddenly, the words stopped flowing. I tried blame the people for whom I was working at the time, but I knew that was only part of the problem. I just couldn't figure it out. In the end, I decided I must simply have run out of gas, that maybe it had something to do with age.

How did I feel about this? one social worker asked. Simple: I felt destroyed. Bereft. As if I had lost something essential to my wellbeing and to my very nature—which I had.

Over the last couple of years, I've learned a lot about my strange disease. I've also regained a modicum of my writing ability (or would like to think so), at least enough to feel up to undertaking this shared attempt to describe the advent of LBD in our lives. I'm not sure if anyone out there will share my opinions, but for now I feel pleased. I can't earn a living as a writer anymore; I know that. But not being the breadwinner doesn't bother me as much as it once had. Many men in their seventies aren't playing that role anymore, in any case.

I have a few thoughts about how things have been going lately. Those peculiar dreams affect me most: they seem to grow longer, longer, and longer. It can take me a full half hour, maybe more, to bring my head back to the present. Often, I can't tell what is a waking dream and what is a whole new "dream set." I patrol the house in the middle of the night, trying to figure out where I am and how I got there. I begin to think that every room in the house is identical, that no matter what room I enter, it will be like every other one. But then I will notice some small object—a book, a bed corner—that contradicts the that assumption. I don't know how to proceed.

All I can do is remind myself not to bump up against the bed because I might knock things off the night table (a lamp, a glass of water, an old mug filled with pencils), or misjudge the distance and go flying across the top of the bed only to land in a heap on the floor on the other side. That's happened twice; once Julie heard the crash, once she didn't. By this time, she had taken to sleeping in another room because both Julie and the family doctor think she needs more sleep. I'm afraid of wearing her down physically, that too many of my late nights may erode her not-so-great reservoir of strength.

Sometimes I overreact to a situation and tiptoe right up to the edge of not knowing anything—where I am, whom I'm with, where we are going. Once, when Julie was late getting home, I panicked and called the police. They didn't seem to take it all that seriously over the phone, but they sent someone over anyway. He was a good man, that officer, a man who knew his job. He calmed me down and made me realize I had better listen to people who know their business. A few minutes later, sure enough, Julie came whistling up the front walk, just as he had predicted.

And more than a year after my first visit to St. Christopher

House, I am still attending the Day Program once a week. After I won the weekly bingo grand prize three weeks in a row—I wasn't even paying attention—the amount of under-the-breath growling from the other clients indicated that I had been accepted as one of the gang. One of these days, I suppose I'll move on, but it will be with a certain amount of regret.

I've been thinking about death a lot lately. Singers Tommy Makem and the last Clancy Brother, Liam, died within a few months of each other last year, and their deaths moved me deeply. Their group had created one of the great sounds of the early Sixties, a mixture of Irish mournfulness and New York élan. They had a sound that was absolutely unique, both profound and poignant at the same time. Julie and I used to sit in the White Horse Tavern listening to them and joining in ourselves, and it seems incredible to me to think that they're all dead and gone now: two in the 1990s, two this year at the way-too-early age of seventy-five. If they can die, and take that music with them, anybody can.

The last time we heard any of the Clancy Brothers was in the late 1980s when we took in a solo concert given by Liam in Cornwall, Ontario. I thought briefly of going up to say hello after the show, but we were with some people and didn't get around to it. We thought we'd catch him next time, whenever that was. It never happened.

It's strange to already know the way I am going to die. Though I can't tell you where or when, I can probably tell you how.

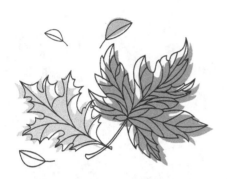

Part II

The People in the Hall

CHAPTER 9

2010

Julie

One snowy evening in February, Ken and I sit around watching a documentary in which a Haitian midwife manages, with considerable skill, to slide safely into the world a baby whose umbilical cord is wrapped around its neck. The scene jogs Ken's memory. He says, "That was me, remember?"

The experts caution people *not* to "reality orient," not even when a dementia sufferer says something wildly inaccurate. I understand the thinking behind the rule, but there are times when it's hard to resist, especially if you played a major role in the memory.

"No, that was John, remember?" I say carefully. "John was the baby. The doctor told us afterward that it was touch and go for a while. You were really worried. Lucky for us, it all turned out well."

"Oh, yes," Ken says. "John was the baby; I was the *mother*."

The confusion and flashes of paranoia that occasionally accompany LBD have picked up speed over the winter. How much should I attribute to the season (the short daylight hours, the bitter cold, the snowstorms that sometimes keep us indoors), and how much to physiology (the good dopamine decreasing as the clumps of abornmal protein increase)? Does it even matter? All I know is that Ken was increasingly insistent on being The Man, the self-appointed micromanager of our daily lives, and I have no choice but to accept it.

"Have you got the others up yet?" he asks, even when there's no one except us in the house.

"Make sure you take *all* of your pills today," he reminds, though my only daily medication is a single tablet for high blood pressure.

"What time do you see the dentist? You don't want to be late," he says, despite the fact the appointment was weeks ago.

When people inquire politely about how Ken is doing, I manage a few words about how he "looked" or "seemed" that week. It's not hedging: as close as we have been for so many years (and in some hard-to-define way still are), I don't know what goes on in his head now. At least, not often. Before he became sick, I always had some idea of what was bothering him—usually something to do with work or an upcoming visit from his parents. But now I wonder if he has any real sense of who I am. Does he know how much his/my/our life has changed lately? Does he remember what our children and grandchildren are up to? Does he know what's going on in the larger world?

Answer came there none. I can study his face all I want; I can observe, listen, and try to understand, but beyond the occasional fleeting smile or flash of anger, it's anyone's guess. And I *hate* this increasing distance between us.

I was in high school when my Grandma Macfie moved in with my family. South African Dutch by birth, she must have been a feisty young woman. When the Boer War broke out, she left her family down on the Cape and made her way to Johannesburg, to hire on as a nurse in, of all places, a British military hospital. One of the enemy, a wounded Scot fighting on the British side, would become my grandfather.

Before coming to live with us, she had already had a couple of falls. Gradually, as her health declined, she stopped going out and eventually took to her bed. She accepted her lot with amazing equanimity, I thought, and it seemed hard when it was my turn to empty her commode that she should feel the need to apologize profusely.

Those years with Grandma were my first hands-on experience of caregiving. Later, as an adult, and with Ken's help, I would nurse our children through a mix of childhood ailments and accidents—chickenpox, mumps, pleurisy, scarlet fever, pneumonia, a bruised spleen, a broken collarbone, two tonsillectomies, two or three concussions. We also served as foster parents to two Korean girls brought to Canada for heart surgery and a Belarus teenager suffering from the lingering effects of Chernobyl. More recently Ken and I had co-authored a television series on health practitioners who combine western medicine with such "alternative" techniques as herbs and massage.

So you would think that with this background I would manage better. But none of it seems to have prepared me for some aspects of this shape-shifting tsunami of a disease.

In collaborating, as in other things, Ken and I have always been frank with each other. One day, while we are at work on this book, I muse out loud to him, "You know, it occurs to me there can't be many people in the world who are writing

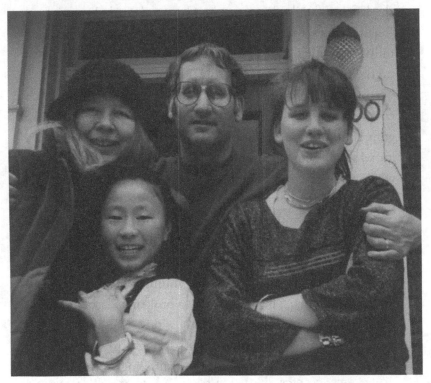

Montreal, 1986: Ken and Julie with their daughter Jane and 12-year-old Korean heart patient Mi Ae, who was in their care while awaiting surgery at Montreal Children's Hospital. Surgeons donated their time so that Mi Ae, and a number of other kids, could return to Korea with healthy hearts.

partners with someone who has dementia." He didn't look the least bothered by my observation, only thoughtful.

"You should put that in," he said.

So I do.

Ken wants very much to keep on writing, or trying to, for as long as he can, and I feel the same way. Yet it's a struggle. The work we've done together so far has been a source of shared pleasure, but this piece isn't just another book; it's our life. With his short term-memory going, it's becoming impossible for him to retain any sense of the manuscript's structure. He will pick up a page, sit reading and rereading, jot down a few indecipherable notes, then drop the page and wander off. Later, after he awakens from his nap, he remembers nothing of what he wrote an hour or two earlier.

Before we began working together, Ken had a long, successful writing career of his own. Supporting a family on freelance work wasn't easy, but a fanciful imagination and robust sense of humor fed into writing for children, while an interest in history and social issues found an outlet in journalism—political columns, film reviews, travel writing. When work dried up in one area, he could shift gears and look for something in the other.

By the mid-Sixties, when a cousin by the name of Herb Klynn offered him an apprenticeship in his small animation studio in Los Angeles, Ken had published several picture books for young kids and was an experienced reporter for the *Village Voice*. On our arrival in California, however, he found the high-ups of network television didn't share the laissez-faire attitude of Dan Wolf, the *Voice* editor famous for printing his contributors' pieces with not so much as a syllable altered.

In Hollywood, no matter what the film genre, frequent plot and dialogue rewrites were considered an integral part of the writing process.

For years afterward, Ken used to speak with admiration about the staff writer assigned to guide him through the basics of story structure. "Tom Dagenais was one patient guy," he told me more than once. "He must have been patient because I was one recalcitrant pupil—but Tom stuck with me, or we stuck with each other. I really learned a lot from him."

Those early lessons in writing for television paid off after our move to Canada. Under the aegis of Ruth Vernon, head of children's programming at TVOntario, the new provincial network, Ken turned out one award-winning series after another. Adults who grew up watching shows Ken wrote wax nostalgic today in the blogosphere about that innovative era in children's television, which spanned twenty years. DVDs of his Readalong series, whose puppet cast included a genial work boot, a talking house, a skeleton, and a pink wedgie shoe named Pretty, continue to be watched by schoolkids and English as a Second Language students in countries around the world. (A French version of the show was hosted by a yellow *ananas formidable* who bantered with a rock group named *Les Squellettes*.)

A series called *Under the Umbrella Tree* for the Canadian Broadcasting Corporation (CBC) ran for seven years. Ken wrote most of the scripts. He received a personal blessing from Astrid Lundgren to pen scripts for Nelvana Animation's Pippi Longstocking series. TVO, however, was in a sense his home; his work there expanded to include documentaries and adult programs such as *Media Circus*, a live TV show about TV.

This innovative series, which Ken also co-hosted, featured cross-network linkups with hosts of other live shows and interviews with such forward-thinkers as Marshall McLuhan and Northrop Frye. Ken's gig at TVOntario was great for the network and for us.

The first time Ken tossed a handful of typed pages in my direction and said brusquely, "You'll probably hate this, but give it a read," took place shortly after our move to New York in 1959. I read his short story and didn't hate it: I was impressed. There is something appealingly audacious about words that until now have never been set down on paper in that particular combination; but in the heightened setting of Greenwich Village, with its offbeat bookshops, late-night jazz clubs, and the new coffeehouses that were opening up all over the place, the uneven black-on-white inkiness of the pages in my hand had an almost electric charge. Since childhood I had derived great pleasure from good writing, and I could recognize talent when I saw it.

All of which I attempted to articulate to Ken that day, at the same time providing what I viewed as a few helpful criticisms of his work. He at first expressed disappointment at my failure to provide complete and utter adoration, but then (typically) he laughed and told me he liked my frank comments. That pattern, set early on in our relationship—him handing me a few pages ("You'll probably hate this…"), me giving my reactions and sometimes jotting a few sentences in the margins—continued over the next three decades, even with the arrival of three babies within five years and our many moves.

A couple of friends with strong feminist leanings expressed dismay at my lifestyle, but we aren't all required to live by the same model. Though I wasn't ready to pursue a career at that point, I enjoyed being around someone who was working hard at having one. I liked being a full-time mother, and the fact that Ken worked at home meant he was available for babysitting when I wanted to get out for a few hours to take music courses or do volunteer work in local schools.

Perhaps it was inevitable, however, that once our youngest child was off to university, we would experiment with co-writing. I was raised in a writing household, falling asleep at night to the *tap-tap-tap* of my father's old Woodstock as he typed out another book on local history or a letter to the editor of *Newsweek* on some current issue. My mother, a fan of the poets Browning and Longfellow, kept a small leather-bound volume handy in which she jotted down her own poems.

At the beginning of my freshman year at Oberlin, my English comp professor had surprised me by reading one of my papers out loud as an example of what the rest of the class should be striving for. This unexpected honor did wonders for my confidence, which was in need of boosting because I had just received an abysmally low mark on a big European history exam. And if fate was sending me a message, I was listening. Over the next four years, I became a master of the three-page essay and avoided like the plague any course that might demand all-night cramming sessions. I also signed on as a feature reporter for the bi-weekly *Oberlin Review* and briefly considered going into journalism, but for the first time in her life, my troubled older sister, who would later be diagnosed with schizophrenia, was moving up the ladder at a daily Chicago-area newspaper; I didn't want to steal her hard-won thunder.

That was then. Since those student days, I had witnessed so many changes, in our personal lives and in the larger world: sit-ins and bus-ins; "Black is beautiful;" gay rights, native rights, and the women's movement; miniskirts; political assassinations; Vietnamese boat people; Pol Pot; color TV; cable; the arrival of the Internet and the instant miracle of email; economic booms and busts; the births of children and grandchildren; our immigration to Canada; the deaths of our parents; career and health issues, including ageing and all that word implies. Also, for the first time in my life, I was reading a lot of history.

My story about enjoying Ken's tales of the Iroquois Confederacy on our first date was never intended as just one more "cute" meeting anecdote, Woody-Allen style. In high school, a one-semester course in Michigan history had made me aware of how much native culture was already familiar to me in the form of street and county names—Erie, Huron, Wyandotte, Tecumseh, Pontiac, Petosky, Muskegon, Genessee, and so many more. Ken took that awareness one step further. He was ahead of his time, as were the educators who made that high school subject a required course. Now, it seemed, every aspect of human life, no matter how local or how universal—the role of landscape on culture, the effect of war on civilian life, sports, history, health, entertainment, housework—was deemed of interest if written about intelligently. I liked this reversal of the old top-down approach to history, which had emphasized kings and queens and famous battles.

The move to the countryside was the catalyst. Leaving the urban for the rural world was a new kind of adventure for us. As a child I had enjoyed the days my family spent at the farms of two uncles, one in Georgia and one in Michigan, but waking up every morning on your own ten-acre piece of land, land that was fronted by a rural route and that sloped down to a gurgling river in back, was a different sort of thing than visiting relatives for a few days. The quiet that surrounded our handyman's bargain was a palpable, living quiet. You could almost *hear* the plants growing. We became intensely aware of the implications of the daily weather report, and in this different environment, with tractors rumbling past the house at all hours and neighbors who talked of crops and tree lots and the high number of pesky deer in the back field this year, we were in the mood to try something new.

One day, when I returned home and told Ken about an article I had come across in a magazine called *Canadian Geographic*, which had been lying around the doctor's waiting room, he proposed we try working on an idea for a piece. I was the one who fished the crumpled pages out of the wastebasket where he hurled them after the editor sent a rejection letter calling our piece "too hokey," too this, too that. When our revised version of the article was finally published in the magazine, more opportunities to work together soon followed.

For me, working with Ken signaled the start of a valued late-life career; for him, it quite literally offered a move into pastures green. There were so many subjects just begging to be written about here in the country: the death and life of small town newspapers, home-styled museums set up in back-road bedrooms, "fence viewers" (local farmers hired to adjudicate in testy boundary disputes), and the continuing popularity of country auctions as an economic form not far removed from the barter system. The last of these subjects provided a chance, on drowsy summer afternoons, to mingle with local people and reflect on their family histories through whatever old belongings were on display. A side benefit was being able to furnish our house, bit by bit, at our leisure, and with minimal cost.

After *Canadian Geographic* printed two of our pieces in one issue, Ken announced that it was time for a book. I wasn't so sure. At this point, we were living in the Beaches area of Toronto, sharing a small office with a single computer, and as a first-time grandparent, I didn't want to lose out on things like walks along the boardwalk with Julian waving hello to the seagulls from his stroller. Also, I pointed out, a book carries a lot more psychological weight than a 2,500-word magazine piece.

Ken listened to my doubts. "I understand what you're saying," he assured me, "but it will be all right. We'll manage." And, except for the time (never repeated) when we made the mistake of working through an entire weekend without a break, he was right. The writing, under the aegis of a sympathetic editor, went well. The book was published to mixed reviews. A second book did better; it got raves on both sides of the border and even made a profit.

Ken's first reaction to his diminishing writing skills had been to blame it on his hearing. The specialist who tested him told him to go home and stop worrying: his hearing was perfect.

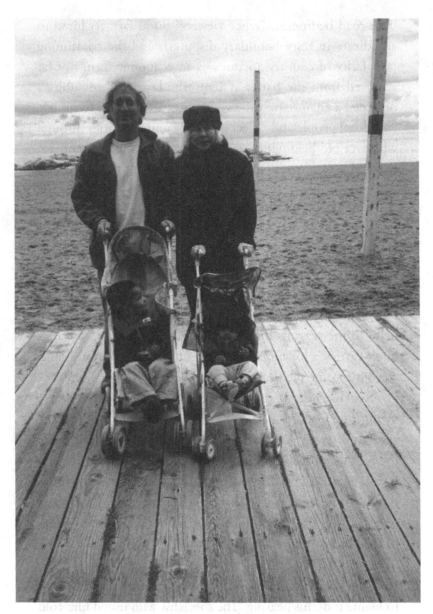

Toronto boardwalk, 1995: Ken and Julie enjoying the fresh air and the seagulls with their first grandchildren, Julian and Elliot.

Later, after the hallucinations began, he became convinced the trouble lay in his vision but, again, was told there was no problem. His instincts were not completely off, though. Artists depend on their observation of the outside world for raw material. Writers and painters make connections, draw conclusions, and toss ideas this way and that. Eventually, the end product is new and meaningful material—or so they hope.

When a social worker asked Ken early on how he felt his diminishing ability to write, he had answered, "It's simple: I feel destroyed. Bereft. As if I had lost something essential to my wellbeing and to my very nature." No wonder the first signs of fuzziness in his brain had thrown him into a tailspin. Vincent van Gogh's madness—or whatever the problem was—didn't make him a better painter; it just meant he had to work harder, and in the end, he shot and killed himself in the middle of a cornfield. Ken's despair at the decline of his creative powers was less extreme than van Gogh's, but probably not by much.

Creative concerns aside, there are practical issues that hinder Ken's writing. The worsening tremor has turned the computer into an ongoing nightmare, especially because mistakes take so long to correct. And since neither of us can read his shaky handwriting, pen and paper are no longer an option. Our kind family doctor has offered us new speech-activated software, but Ken told him, "Thanks, but my voice is so soft now. And I keep forgetting words. It just wouldn't work."

Ken is probably right. A while back, the LBDA website announced plans for a forum devoted exclusively to patients.

It sounded like a good idea, but the number of dementia sufferers who signed up to participate was minute compared to the never-ending torrent of probing, confiding, worrying, advising emails from caregivers on their forum. Patients evidently found the idea of organizing their scattered thoughts and sending them out into cyberspace rather daunting; it's not surprising that a former psychiatrist ("former" because his symptoms forced an early retirement) is among the few who have joined the online conversation.

The Knitting Doc (the psychiatrist's web name) writes about the difficulty people with LBD have with words:

> "Whenever a word won't come, [I] picture a long tunnel starting at the front of my head, progressing to the back of my head…. At the back, sometimes there is nothing there, thus no word. At other times, there is a vague dot or small object or small word [that] is incomprehensible. Sometimes, I can visualize [the word] slowly coming to the front of the tunnel. How far it comes up seems to determine whether I get the word. Sometimes, I literally pause and wait for it to come forth. Sometimes, it will only come halfway and then stop. This is actually more frustrating than if it is just totally blocked. Other times… the right word [comes] but in slow motion. That's when I find myself talking and literally saying, 'Wait a minute…'"

The Knitting Doc's confession helps shed some light on Ken's communication challenges. After taking another look at the job of writing about our experience with LBD, we settle on a new plan, one that I hope will, in the words of The Knitting Doc, help Ken "move his thoughts to the front of his head." We've both done lots of interviewing; now I would try interviewing him on whatever subject was running through his mind, take down his words and type them up for him to edit when and if he feels ready.

Ken is eager to try.

"Something new this winter," he begins one afternoon, as I sit nearby with a legal pad and pile of sharpened pencils. "I call it my morning disappearances. There's a long period after I first get up—it can seem as much as two hours, though it is probably much less or maybe more—when I have no sense of where I am or even *who* I am. When I wake up in someone else's head, or at least it feels like that. Things look familiar, but I don't feel as if I'm there. When Julie tries to convince me that I'm in my own house, it takes time, but at some point I tell her I've come out of it. At first, I'm not really out of it even though I say I am. Then, eventually, I look around and see it is true. I *am* in my own house. It can take her perhaps half an hour to convince me things are as she says they are."

A good start. I type it up and hand him a printout, saying, "When you want to do some more, let me know." But this first attempt proves a false dawn. The next few times we try, he is so embarrassed by his long pauses after a lifetime of being able to quickly hit on the right words that it seems cruel even to raise the issue. Day by day, the confusion is winning out.

But I have one other source for continuing the story:

the notes I have been keeping since the LBD diagnosis. I am acutely aware of the responsibility I will be taking on if we continue with the project. Ken is so vulnerable these days; his cognition flickers like a light bulb about to burn out. I will have to write every sentence with that fact in mind.

I'm also concerned that if we continue to work together, it may add another level of guilt to my feeling of being always in the wrong. No one has expressed the caregiver's dilemma as well as Russian writer Lidiya Ginzburg. In her book *Blockade Diary*, she describes watching her sick, elderly mother slowly starve to death during the nine-hundred-day seige of Leningrad. For the sick person, Ginzburg points out, the order of daily experience is meaningless, but "for the person standing nearby and bearing the guilt and responsibility," there is a constant need to "construct the life of the other."

In all my attempts to help Ken make sense of his life, I am haunted by guilt no matter what choices I make. When I push him into attending the day program, I feel wrong, even though he enjoys it once he's there. But when I give in to his grumbling and cancel, leaving him free to stare at CNN all day, I feel equally bad. When the geriatrician asks, "How do *you* think your husband is doing?" it seems just plain rude to speak in the third person about someone sitting an arm's length away; but if I wait until Ken is asleep to phone the doctor and give him a fuller report, that feels like telling tales. When on rare occasions I correct Ken on some small question of fact—like the story of the midwife—I end up feeling churlish. However, following the do-not-confront rule religiously is such a doctrinaire approach that it makes me uncomfortable.

Somewhere, even with dementia, there has to be room for life to enter between the cracks.

In the end, I tell myself that there's an important story to be told. I aso remind myself that Ken, once committed to any project, has always prided himself on completing it. He wouldn't want me to be hobbled by doubts.

I agree to continue—making sure that in doing so I speak as carefully for him as I am for myself, and, with the help of quotes from my note-taking, letting him speak as much as possible in his own words.

CHAPTER 10

One morning, Ken wakes me at six with an urgent request: "Get up, I need you. Hurry. I can't find my keys." What I call his waking dreams and what he calls his "morning disappearances" make this time of day a special challenge. I've never been a morning person and over the course of the night, somewhere deep inside my mouth, a toothache has announced itself. My mumbled, "later, maybe?" is not an acceptable answer.

Off we head on another of our lost key safaris, a familiar route around the apartment. No keys in their designated home on top of the tall bookcase. No keys on the kitchen counter or in the bathroom drawer where he keeps his shaving things. No keys on the bedside table. I'm running out of places to look. I check various jackets and plunge my hands deep into the pockets of his green cargo pants, but they come up empty. We lift up newspapers and look in various nooks and crannies. I have an extra set put away somewhere, but Ken wants his own keys.

By the time I spot his key ring with the hockey logo, mixed in with the tangled heap of my jewelry on the dresser, I am feeling a bit testy myself. Taking a couple of deep breaths, I remind myself that there's no point in asking why anyone except the head housekeeper of the Grand Hotel would be looking for house keys at this hour. As I fill the kettle for his tea, there is a brief moment when, for the first time, I realize that I could answer "yes!" to the unspoken question that has occasionally hovered over us: should we start thinking about long-term care?

No, not yet, I tell myself. *I'm not ready; we're not ready.*

That night at dinner he puts down his fork and asks, "Can you see me?"

He is serious. I assure him that I can see him clearly.

"Good!"

We go back to our chicken curry.

The morning after the night before, after a late night enjoying the sight of skiers, bobsledders, and lugers in the Vancouver Olympics repeatedly plunge downhill at terrifying angles in search of "owning the podium," we are both experiencing TV hangovers. Ken is especially hard hit.

"I don't know where I am. What is this place?" he asks me. "Did all the Canadian teams lose?"

March 1: The neurologist has started him on a new drug— one half of a Lilliputian-sized pill called Seroquel. *If* it helps control Ken's increasing agitation (as it has done for many), the doctor will increase the dosage. He might also then consider increasing the Levocarb in the hope of reducing the stiffness and tremor. (Levocarb improves the flow of dopamine in the brain; without the right amount of dopamine, it's as if a brake keeps going on when you attempt to move your body. At an advanced stage of the disease, patients may find themselves stuck halfway up a flight of stairs, unable to go forward or back.)

Unfortunately for Ken, *if* doesn't turn into *when*. Twelve hours after the first dose, I find him standing in the dark hall looking as if there were no *there* there, or anywhere else, for that matter. When I speak he doesn't answer. I take him by the hand and lead him slowly back to the bedroom. He goes willingly, but once there he just continues to stand silent and rigid. Finally, I leave a small light on and return to my own bed. Eventually he will lie down, won't he? The only other option is to phone for an ambulance or wake Corry or Jane out of a sound sleep and ask for help; so far I've managed to avoid both those alternatives. In the meantime, at least one of us will get some sleep.

In the morning, I go to check on him. Sure enough, he's out cold. Around ten, when he eventually gets up, he tells me he's fine, so good that he's going to walk down to College Street for an infusion of household cash. I've spoken with the staff at the bank, and the tellers know to keep an eye on him. He may not be out and about on his own much longer, and I know these few remaining interactions with the larger world matter greatly to him.

"I'm a bit shaky," he admits on his return. "There I was standing in the line, and suddenly I forgot who I was. I didn't know my own name. Can you imagine? I was in a panic until I thought of my wallet. My driver's license had my name on it: Ken Sobol. I was okay then."

I congratulate him on his display of practical thinking. It feels like another of those small victories, one that we can enjoy together. Evidently he's still "there" sometimes.

Still, I phone the neurologist. We decide to drop the Seroquel for now.

March 8: John is here from Ottawa for a few days. After dinner he picks up the guitar, as he often does on these visits, tries a few chords, and over the next hour or so the three of us sing our way through a free-associating inter-generational repertoire. When we reach back to Dylan's "Masters of War," though bit rusty on some of the verses, Ken joins in full force on the chorus and John smiles.

Father and son have clashed occasionally in recent years (mostly on Ken's side), but now some unfathomable shift in mood has taken place and John is back in his good books. The other day, when it had been longer than usual between visits, he told me, "I *miss* John." As a mother, this is music to my ears, as welcome as a new Dylan song.

Two days later and Ken is repeatedly claiming that there are two identical—but different—houses, and *we are in the wrong one.* As early as 2008, after attending a choir party in the suburbs, he had described to me the odd sensation of being in two places at the same time. "It's something like a double exposure," he had said. "Our house but with the one belonging to Marg and Don sort of superimposed."

There have been occasional repeats of that pattern since then, but Ken has always accepted it if I told him something like, "That might have been a dream, because right now we're at home as usual, in our own house." This time the fuzziness about which house we're in lingers. I resort to pointing to our familiar artwork hanging on the walls, our benign beige sofa sitting at its place in front of the window, our pile of Times Literary Supplements on the table waiting to be read. Nothing helps. By afternoon, he is starting to move on, but his agitation in the meantime has been distressing to watch.

Four days later and the "wrong" house obsession has lasted all day. He is so upset, and I desperately want to help, but no words are the right words. This sudden downward lurch is hard to handle when I am back and forth to various dental specialists for a root canal, gum surgery, and a new crown. I have to ask someone to stay with him on these occasions or at least, over his repeated objections, drop in to check that everything is alright.

I've also just started a second course of antibiotics for a lingering virus. On the streetcar, people move discreetly but quickly away when one of my coughing fits really gets going. This prescription had better work. I am caregiver to two people in this house, and I can't do a good job (I tell myself huffily) with Ken's considerable needs if I don't pay some attention to my own regime. I need time to do the daily tai chi set; the boring but essential back exercises for degenerative disc disease; the frequent checking of my blood pressure; the daily eye drops; and the nasal lavages and brews of mullein tea when I feel a sinus infection coming on. Most annoying of all my own problems is the ever-present hum of tinnitus.

One morning, there's an atypically plaintive tone to Ken's voice when he comes into the kitchen.

"I don't understand what I'm supposed to do next. What do I do?" he asked.

Until this moment, he has always preferred to get his own breakfast.

"Some food would be a good thing, right?" I volunteer, trying unsuccessfully to sound upbeat. He stands to one side, watching silently as I take down a dish and get out the milk and cereal. "Here's your cereal—here on the table. Come and eat."

He sits down, arms stiff at his sides. "What do I do next?" he asks. "I don't know what you mean."

"Just pick up the spoon. Take a bite," I urge. "You like this kind: Ancient Grains." He obeys and then immediately sets down the spoon. "Good. Try another one," I encourage.

He turns to look up at me, puzzled. "Isn't there a picture with it? I thought there might be a tattoo there."

A childhood memory of cereal box prizes? But now he has picked up the spoon again and is digging in.

It's such a relief to see him emerge from one of these waking dreams, to watch his face transmute itself, sometimes within seconds, from a bamboozled blankness to a bright look of being in the here and now. I've never gotten used to it. Each time, I feel I am witnessing a miracle, a reverse version of the main character's transmutation in an old Wolfman movie or, to use a happier simile, like seeing the sky brighten in the East after a long, restless night.

When the minibus arrives at ten to ferry him to his weekly day program, I'm feeling wrung out and the day has only just begun. Once the bus helper has escorted him safely on board and I've waved good-bye, I pick up the phone. Corry suggests he begin spending one day a week at their place. We've discussed this possibility before, but stairs are a worry at Corry and Greg's since the bedrooms and the bath are on the second floor. So far the few falls Ken has experienced have not resulted in any major injuries—but he's been lucky.

"Tell you what, Mom. Why don't I invite him to go for a drive this afternoon instead?" she asks. "Maybe a change of scene will help. He usually likes that, right?"

I'm happy to accept the offer. As I've learned more about the disease, I've tried to minimize dependence on other people, but this morning's confusion has revealed a new, disturbing level of disorientation.

Author Tom Kitwood, a British psychologist who for years has worked with dementia sufferers and their caregivers, writes:

> Those who have this role take on, almost single-handed, a colossal task. The weight of evidence from anthropology is that no individual was ever "designed" for such an onerous commitment; human beings emerged through evolution as a highly social species, where burdens are carried by a group.... [The] process of dementia is also the story of a tragic inadequacy in our culture.

If it sounds self-serving to say I agree with him, so be it. My belief is that, just as we all set out to be good parents (even if we're all doomed to partial failure in the attempt), we also have an innate desire to do right by any family member who develops a serious disease. Even dementia. Or especially dementia. It's not just child-raising that requires a village. Caregiving can't be learned in isolation; you crave the reassuring presence of others who are going through the same thing and the advice of people who have already been there.

I find watching the zeitgeist unfold endlessly entertaining. I have no desire to go back to the past, any part of the past. To paraphrase Dr. Johnson, if you don't enjoy the present era, you must be tired of life itself. But every age brings its challenges, and Kitwood has put his finger on one of ours. In the twenty-first century, the village that's needed to help raise a child, or guide a teenager through the ups and downs of adolescence, or care for a senior with acute dementia, is a very, very busy village indeed.

There are so many demands on the energies of villagers and so little time to sit and stare, observe, and just "be." Each day brings with it new social issues to sort out, new technologies to get used to. Women no longer chat with neighbors over the clothesline; modern men don't often hang out at the corner barbershop. We work, work, work, and when we're not working, we're busy helping the kids with their homework or trying to figure out the instruction book for the latest electronic gadget we've bought with the money from all that overtime. Having an occasional hour free for contemplation is a basic human need, as necessary as food and water, and we're all starved for it.

Ken is more willing to listen to the younger generation than to me when someone must take on the authority role. "Dad," Corry tells him over lunch one day in late March, "you know that Mom's bronchitis hasn't gone away yet, right? And you know the doctor says she needs more rest."

He nods reluctantly. "Well," she continues, "I've been talking with May, your new case worker at the CCAC." (In Ontario, the local Community Care Access Centre is the provincial body responsible for supervising eligibility and admission into long-term care residences.)

He gives another nod. "Okay. She's coming to see you tomorrow. She thinks you may be eligible for a short-term stay in a nursing home—you know, just a few days to give Mom a break. One of the places you've already visited."

The next morning, Ken is very subdued. I had been busy at the computer for awhile when, getting on to noon, I suddenly notice that it is unusually quiet in the house. When I open the bedroom door, I see Ken, curled in fetal position, sound asleep, wearing his spiffy new spring jacket over a nightshirt and a new pair of Levis. In what for him must be turbulent times, he needs touchstones; these items are favorites—an adult version of a toddler's security blanket.

March 23: Yesterday afternoon, when he complained that there were several things missing from his wallet, I opened it to show him that everything was intact. A small scrap of paper fluttered out. Picking it up off the rug, I could just decipher the three words: wallet, keys, glasses. His reminder of essentials to keep close at hand in a world that includes social workers, day programs, and uncomfortable phrases like "short-term care."

Today, after his nap, I tell him, "You look rested, you must have had a good sleep."

"Yeah, except for that guy I had to beat up."

"Oh, you mean a dream?"

"No, he was real."

The distinction between lucidity and confusion is increasingly blurred.

At two on the dot, the doorbell rings. It's the CCAC rep with Corry coming up the walk behind her. May, whom I've met only over the phone, turns out to be a tiny woman with an early pregnancy bump and a direct, easy manner. I take to her right away, and I can see Ken likes her, too. He is putty in her hands as, without any preamble, she launches into a frank discussion of the advancing state of his disease and reminds him that caregivers, like everyone else, need their share of rest. By the time she leaves, he has agreed to a week in mid-May at Wellesley Central Residence.

March 27: A while back, Ken declared in his oracle-like way, "You'll soon be married to some rich guy."

"I'm living with the guy I love," I told him. "And where do you get these ideas, anyway?"

"I get them from my imagination," he said.

The next morning, before I've even put my feet on the floor, he casually declares, "I noticed you had someone else in bed with you last night." He studies my face while I protest that I've been alone all night. He tells me, "I believe you."

If I describe any of his more outré symptoms to people and they remind me that "it's just the illness talking," my grouchy—though usually unspoken—reaction is, "But that doesn't keep the sound of the words from hurting."

Early on, one young social worker, listening to my self-doubt about coping with the many moods of LBD, reminded me that it's *because* I'm the most important person in Ken's life that I have become the target of his negative emotions. She meant to be encouraging, and perhaps there is some truth to her words. But isn't that the kind of thing they used to say to excuse wife beaters?

CHAPTER 11

After a wakeful night, I'm up early on a prematurely warm spring morning. The radio weatherman is beside himself with excitement about a predicted high of 22 degrees Celsius.

When Ken gets up, he surprises me by apologizing for keeping me awake last night. Even though it wasn't an especially wakeful night, his words are welcome. Like a lot of men, he has done his fair share of saying he's "sorry" over the years. (One of his favorite rock hits used to be "Sorry," which he sang as he walked around the house: "I ran all the way home / chachacha, chachacha / just to say I'm sorry / chachacha, chachacha / What more could I say / chachacha, chachacha / I ran all the way-ay-ay / yay yay yay yay yay.") But now it's my turn to say "I'm sorry" when there's any kind of disagreement. Since he's in a good mood, however, this seems like a good opportunity to tell him about the second part of my two-pronged plan for getting some rest. I've been putting it off for too long.

"Remember that place on Baldwin, the inn where we stayed when our bedroom on Grace Street was being painted?" I ask over breakfast, using my zen breathing to stay focused as I begin to talk about my hunger for some solid sleep. "I've reserved a room there for two nights: tomorrow and Wednesday," I go on. "While I'm gone, John will come and keep you company. You two can watch all the sports you like. John says he's looking forward to spending some time with you."

He hears me out, and when I'm done, he says cheerfully, "I'm glad you explained that for me."

I hug him. A good moment, I think.

By night, he is frantic for me to find the Raptors game on TV. He played basketball in high school and still loves the sport. Aside from the pure entertainment value of the fast play, he is taken away to a safer era while he watches the game. It's not on any of the three sports channels, but I locate the announcer's excited shouts on an AM radio station. Ken stands close to the set, leaning over it, and listening intently. Thank goodness the Raptors win the game.

In the middle of the night, Ken experiences a new house worry: "I've been in another house, the one belonging to that criminal brother-in-law, or whatever he is. And it's your fault! You were the one who was supposed to show me the way home." I have no idea what it is I have done or left undone. And who is the mysterious brother-in-law? Our only relatives in Canada are our son and daughters and their families.

Thursday, April 1, the big day. My first break since the arrival of LBD, and I'm having last-minute doubts. The waiter at Café Diplomatico looked uneasy yesterday after he set down our cappuccinos and Ken told him, with a glare, *"Finally! I thought I would have to come find you and knock you down."* Will he and John be able to manage?

Many of our recent conversations, when they haven't run to invisible houses or sports events, have involved the imaginary troublemakers he sees hanging around the place—gangs of noisy children, criminal types, cousins he hasn't visited in decades. (He has also begun asking me to change the channel whenever a violent scene comes on.) During John's last visit, Ken woke him at three a.m. to ask, "Who are all those people with flashlights coming at me?"

He has even moved our easy-going upstairs neighbors, over to the dark side. "I don't know how they're doing it," Ken tells me, "but they are sending down some stuff that's getting all over me! Making my skin itchy! I think they're injecting it into our apartment somehow."

By noon, when John arrives, Ken's mood has improved. You would think that by now, more than two years after the diagnosis, I would remember how fast his moods can change, but it still often happens that I'm one step behind.

"Those small animals are so clever, the way they run around, all the things they can do," he tells John cheerfully. "I noticed that Harriet is even putting them to work in the garden." The fact we had watched Disney's *Snow White* a couple of nights earlier may explain that comment.

John and Ken drop me off at the inn, and as the two of

them turn to wave good-bye from the front seat, I think to myself, *We can do this.*

Home again. Baldwin Street isn't Paris, but after a winter of close confinement to quarters, it proved not a bad substitute. The prematurely warm weather meant I didn't need a jacket as I sat that first day alone, enjoying a glass of beer, like a real adult, on the sunny front patio of an Indian restaurant. My hour of total immersion in a roomful of Rembrandt and Lucien Freud etchings at the Art Gallery of Ontario, just around the corner from the inn, was pure visual pleasure.

At the inn's communal breakfast table, tourists from Europe and Quebec asked for advice from Canadian guests. Where's the best place for Vietnamese food? Do people like the mayor? Should we take the ferry to the Islands or rent a canoe? Is there really an underground city, and where is it? I find myself enjoying the chance to exercise my rusty social skills; between our long sojourn on backcountry roads and the isolating experience of living with Ken's illness, they have suffered.

Once I'm home, I realize that I needn't have worried about John and Ken's ability to cope. After three days away, I find the house still standing, the dishes washed and stacked, the broom hanging in the broom closet.

The next morning, the first thing Ken asks is, "What's happening?" I have to think for a minute before answering; these days, the most innocuous reply to one of his open-ended questions can provoke irritation.

"Not too much," I venture. "It rained last night."

"Well," he says angrily, walking away, "if you're going to keep it to yourself, never mind!"

That evening, his vision questions resurface. "Do you see me?" he turns to me and asks.

"Yes."

"Do you see the cars in the street?"

I try a joke. "Well, I probably would if we opened the curtains."

He nods, pleased.

(John reports another version of the disappearing question. While I was away, Ken asked him, "Do you see my feet?" Again, a look of relief at John's positive answer.)

My respite experiment had gone well, but Ken's continuing deterioration is worrisome enough that we have begun looking into "crisis care," the CCAC's term for any situation when the family is having difficulty managing care at home. There's a Catch-22, though—a big one. If we apply to be considered for crisis care but no bed is available from our list of preferred residences, Ken could end up being housed indefinitely (or until a better place opens up) in an over-crowded building in a dodgy neighborhood or in one of the new places going up in the far outer suburbs of Toronto, the kind that are reached by three different changes of bus.

Everything in my world feels uncertain. I dread what lies ahead: the almost inevitable move to long-term care and all that implies for both of us. It is impossible that to believe that we might soon not be living under the same roof. On August 28, we are due to celebrate our fiftieth anniversary. The younger generation have been hinting at a party, albeit a very low-key one—perhaps just a cake and bottle of wine here at home.

"Dinna worry, dinna fret," I tell myself, reciting the Scottish version of "Keep a stiff upper lip." The simple phrase helps; even dread is to some degree a matter of choice. It's helpful that as Ken's condition becomes more obvious, I get fewer of the "but he can't be ill, he seems just fine" remarks.

We can hold on awhile longer.

CHAPTER 12

April 9: Early this morning, when we meet in the hall, Ken says, "I don't see you. I can't see you."

Later on, I check my voicemail and find that May has left a message: "Mrs. Sobol, a place has just opened up for May 3. Are you interested? Let me know."

I walk down to the café on the corner to make the return call. A high school tour group has chosen this moment for a pit stop, and the noise is deafening, but I find a chair and dial May's number. An aide informs me May is out of the office, but she can be reached. Surrounded by teens discussing the minutiae of their social lives, I sip my cappuccino and debate the pros and cons of May's offer. If an occasional short-term stay were workable, that would ease the pressure I feel—it might even enable Ken to stay at home indefinitely, which is what we both would like. On the other hand, the mere mention of rejigging the date might cause him to change his mind about the whole thing.

My musings are interrupted by a sound not unlike the braying klaxon of ambulances used in some European cities. I have a foolish moment when I look around for the source and realize it's a cellphone ringing; not only that, the sound is coming from inside my purse—it's *my* cellphone. I have to raise my voice to be heard over the din, and don't like conducting sensitive conversations at the top of my lungs, but the kids, busy with their lattes, are quite oblivious. I tell May that I will accept the earlier date, but I turn down her offer to extend the visit from one to two weeks.

At home, Ken exhibits no reaction when I tell him of the change. But later he says, out of the blue, "A week is a long time."

Three days later, we head for our regular eye checkups. I booked us both on the same afternoon, thinking we could manage a simple trip to the optometrist's—a tactical error. The other patients glance over nervously as Ken glowers at them from his seat in the tiny storefront office. One woman's polite attempt to discuss the likelihood of rain is quickly deflected, and the room settles into an awkward silence. When it is Ken's turn, he has trouble maneuvering his chin into position on the headrest of the examination table. Marty takes me aside before we leave and politely suggests that it might be better if I arranged a separate appointment for Ken next time, preferably at some quiet hour in the work day: a reasonable request.

After dinner, we are in the living room together when

Ken glances over. "Do you see Greg sitting over there on the couch? There were lots of people a minute ago, but the rest of them left," he asks.

"No, I don't see Greg. I kind of wish that I could. Maybe then I would better understand what you mean."

He is quiet, waiting for more. "It must be strange for you," I add hesitantly, "but...I suppose it must also be interesting, in a way."

"Yes, it is. It is *interesting*."

It's Tuesday, recycling day—a weekly ritual Ken prides himself on still being able to manage. Around four p.m., he goes outside to wheel the empty containers back to their place down the narrow laneway between our house and the one next door. A few minutes later, I hear a loud knock at the front door. Harriet, whom the landlord hires to keep our front and back gardens presentable, rushes in without waiting.

"Your husband has fallen! He needs an ambulance!"

I grab my jacket and run outside in my bare feet. Ken is seated on the cement walkway between the houses. A neighbor holds a folded towel to the bloody gash on his forehead. Harriet whips off her wool scarf, and wraps it round his neck. In spite of the warm spring, the cold still lingers in the laneway's heavy shade. I put my down jacket around his shoulders and quickly dial 911 with shaky fingers.

Ken, in his last attempt at dictation, later described the incident:

"The recent crash up at side of house. A serious new element has entered the picture. Or maybe it was something I'd been building up to for the past year or so. Anyway, I took a majestic fall—not an ordinary fall, but a stupendous crash the width of our side alley. I tripped on a huge crack in the cement, two or three inches high, over which I was wheeling our garbage cans. Pushing them as hard as I could, I shot across the cans and, with an enormous thunk, smacked my forehead on the drainpipe of the house next door.

"A pregnant pause, and then people sprang into action. A neighbor came pelting from across the street to see what could have happened; a gardener, working just up the alley, joined her. I didn't know whether I was unconscious or not. I couldn't seem to move. By now Julie was there, too, and since they're always telling you to be careful about head injuries, she decided she had better call for an ambulance."

After the ambulance arrives, two paramedics named Isaac and Craig get Ken safely cocooned on a stretcher and I climb in beside him. One of the men suggests adding a neck brace. As we drive, they fire quick questions at me. How's your husband's general health? What are his medications? How much blood has he lost?

Ken is quiet and cooperative during the ride, but once in the hospital as he lies stretched out on a cart in the busy hallway, he begins complaining about the neck brace; he instructs anyone who passes near—whether nurse, doctor, cleaner, or visitor wandering through on their way to the coffee shop—"Get them to speed things up, can't you! I can't stay here all day!" They all ignore him; the ER has its own well-oiled internal logic, as we know from years of watching George Clooney, Hugh Laurie, and their ilk on the small screen.

It isn't really very long before a nurse with an I-think-you'll-live expression appears to check his vitals. A smiling doctor then cleans up the blood, closes the gash with space-age adhesive and tiny strips of tape, and sends Ken for an x-ray. It reveals no serious damage, but we are asked to wait for a CAT scan "just in case." By now, both of our daughters have arrived to keep us company and help us worry. Jane offers to take him upstairs for the scan.

It's getting late. I walk through the eerie half-lit corridors of the huge hospital in search of food. By the time I return with chips and bottled water, Ken and Jane are back. Finally, after a total of five hours on the stretcher, he is told he can remove the brace. I am happy: no concussion, no spinal damage, just the advice to Ken to, "Get some rest, and leave things to heal on their own."

We head out into the night to hail a taxi.

Twenty-four hours later, Ken is prowling the house, talking under his breath. I catch only bits and pieces. "There's going to be a riot...the kids will...(mumble, mumble)...the hotel...(mumble, mumble)...trouble. You are warned."

Warned of what?

Later, it comes out: "I keep thinking you can't wait to put me away."

The accident has shaken him, and maybe me, more than I realized. I hug him and say, "No one wants to put anybody away. But I don't know how long I'll be able to manage on my own. We've talked about all this before; we even visited some of the nursing homes, remember?"

Back in 2008, the summer after the LBD diagnosis, I had looked at some long-term care facilities online. Ken and I were comfortable enough with the idea then; after all, we might not need one of those places for years—maybe never if the hope-springs-eternal "miracle cure" turned up.

When I told Ken I was going to tour some of the facilities and asked if he would like to go along, he'd agreed. As we strolled through the hushed, carpeted public rooms of the first residence, passing wall after wall hung with the portraits of various royals, I was reminded of the fact that, despite Toronto's deserved reputation as the most multi-ethnic city in the world, the "Maple Leaf Forever" days still form a part of its cultural mosaic. The Queen's face stares up at you each time you search through a handful of change for the right coin, and several ornate nineteenth-century buildings downtown remain a stately backdrop to the daily activities of Toronto's residents.

Once we had finished the tour and closed the door behind us, Ken raised his eyes to the sky. "Not here! Never. No, thank you!" he cried.

The second long-term care residence had a livelier feel and was closer to our apartment—a big plus. Unfortunately, it also came with a long waiting list.

The third place, where some visionary had thought to build a playground adjacent to the front lobby for children of the staff, displayed some imaginative cross-generational thinking. The happy shouts of children carried into the bright front lobby where a crowd of seniors was lined up, waiting for ice cream. I almost looked round to see if a promo was being shot, but the good cheer was real.

The fourth residence won my vote, though. It had good light, an inner courtyard with cherry trees in bloom, and generously sized public rooms on the main floor for socializing. Architecture is not the most important element in a care facility, but even the foggiest psyche must benefit from the sense of wellbeing that good architecture imparts. The patients must, at some level, think: If someone built this beautiful structure for my use, I must be deserving of it.

It's so easy to be casual about the distant future. Ken had taken those early tours in stride, but as his symptoms increased, day by day, month by month, he had become less and less comfortable with the idea. One morning, he had announced casually, "I don't think we'll ever need one of those residences. I'll get worse eventually, I suppose, and right at the end, I might have to go to a hospice or something like that. But until then, I think I'll just stay at home." End of conversation.

Today, though, when I remind him that we had been pleasantly surprised by at least three of the places on those early tours he says, "Yes, I do remember. I'll give it a try—for one week."

April 18: This morning Ken's cousin Larry phoned from Los Angeles. As kids growing up in Cleveland, the two had chummed around together at family parties. Later, Larry moved to the West Coast in search of television work; unlike us, once he found it, he and Marilyn stayed on. Since learning about the illness, Larry had phoned often to engage Ken in talking shop and swapping stories about grandchildren. These long-distance conversations had always perked Ken up, but just a couple of minutes into today's call he halts in mid-sentence, then says: "I'm sorry, Larry...I just...I can't...I can't talk any more." He looks defeated as he reaches up and hands me the phone. One more sign that the disease is picking up its pace if he can't enjoy speaking with Larry, one of the kindest of men.

After dinner, a quiet evening with the television off for once. I welcome the silence, but when I put down my book and glance over at Ken, he is looking so morose that I leave my chair, move to the small footstool nearby, and take his hand. Looking up at him, I speak about my stay at the inn earlier this month, about how nervous I was at the thought of meeting new people, about managing to stop worrying about him and just be on my own.

"The break did me good," I say. "Really. And who knows, this week might do the same thing for you, don't you think? Just finding out that you can cope on your own, in a different setting, might make you feel better."

He is quiet for a moment, maybe remembering the time when the doctors told us that the course of LBD is so unpredictable it can go along for years and then suddenly jump to an acute level.

"Maybe you're right," Ken relents. "Maybe it makes sense to try out one of these places now."

A few days later, Ken wakes me at four a.m. to pass on a racing tip: "Seabiscuit is the name of the horse. He's paying eight to one." It's as if he's casting us as characters in a Damon

Runyon short story—short, pithy sentences, a sprinkling of the vernacular.

Does this new verbal quirk reflect some shift in the arrangement of his brain cells? Or is he practicing his conversational skills in anticipation of the upcoming week in short-term care? Trying it on, the way stand-up comics must do when they're working out a new act?

Later, Ken brings in the folded newspaper from the front porch and holds it out to me, commenting, "Promises a lot, fails to deliver." He then asks conversationally, as if the two of us were fellow guests at a seaside watering hole, "What brings you down here?"

"Oh, nothing special," I reply. "I thought I'd just sit for a while and read the paper."

"Any particular subject of interest?"

"Not really. You could give me the front page for a start, I guess."

He hands it over and goes off to get dressed.

April 27: After dinner, I am at the computer, and Ken sits, absorbed, in the Raptors game on TV. When a commercial break comes on, he walks over and asks courteously, as he might of a fellow fan sitting next to him at the game, "Can you tell me where the nearest bathroom is?"

I take him out to the hall and point him in the right direction. "Second door on the right," I say.

A minute later, he comes back. "It's occupied," he says matter-of-factly.

Yet still, from time to time, he can come up with an unexpected insight. After he made a quick transition from dream state to reality early this morning, he told me, "Today I went three times back and forth, but I got out of it faster than before. That's good!"

Yes, it is!

One morning Ken declares himself to be working up for more dictation. By afternoon, he has completely forgotten and seems very uneasy. Every once in a while, he utters a cryptic comment:

"So this is where the big contest takes place? Here, in the living room?"

"Did you notice all those people hanging from hooks in the hall?"

"It really throws me the way people just keep disappearing. Not people we know...I don't know who they are. Sometimes, there'll be two of them talking to me, and then I just turn and they're gone. It's really quite upsetting."

By evening he is complaining about every aspect of his life, including the upcoming short-term stay. I'm casting about for the right thing to say when an image flashes in my mind: the sign I used to contemplate while waiting for Ken in the cancer hospital pharmacy. "The hardest thing in the world is to listen to someone in trouble—and to do it without offering solutions," it read.

So I let him talk away and try to listen and not speak, not judge. He needs the opportunity to express himself so badly; it seems to help.

CHAPTER 13

Sunday, May 2: I've arranged for cable service in Ken's room at Wellesley Central, downloaded a copy of their monthly newsletter, and picked out some family pictures for him to look at if he gets lonely. As I pack his bag, a line from a punchy Randall Jarrell poem Ken used to quote pops into my head:

In folly's mailbox
Still laughs the postcard, Hope:
Your uncle in Australia
Has died and you are Pope.

Still laughs the postcard. Maybe he will profit from the break, I tell myself. He might remember how much he used to enjoy meeting new people (some of whom, in this case, may also be conversationally challenged). He might return home with a bit of his old ready-for-anything self restored.

Wellesley Central is one of the places we toured in 2008, the one with the interior courtyard. It has been a while since the tour, though. We decide to try a quick reconnaissance mission, thinking we'll just drive past the place, but on impulse we park and go inside. Sitting in the courtyard under the blooming cherry trees, Ken appears at ease.

The Monday morning air is blissfully warm, freshened by last night's rain. By ten a.m., with rush hour pretty much over, the short drive takes no time at all. We park in the residence's underground space, sign ourselves in, and locate Ken's private (technically, "semi-private" because he shares a bathroom) third-floor room. While I set out a few photos, the charge nurse and the physiotherapist drop by for a chat. Ken shakes hands with everyone, answers questions, on his best behavior. Everything seems fine.

A staff member comes in to announce lunch and invites me to join him. After the meal, Ken waves me off. "You might as well go now," he says.

Tuesday: So far so good. I sit with Ken again at lunch, marveling at the wait staff's endless pool of patience. The servers approach each client in turn, holding out a tray with a sample of the two mains, standing there while they take their time choosing. One woman at our table shakes her head angrily at everything on offer. "Potato," she answers to every question. The server eventually leaves and returns quickly with a plate of mashed potatoes and salad.

Ken is famous among the grandchildren for two things:

his jokes and his sweet tooth. But chocolate bars, in this health-conscious era, are not on the menu. That's his only complaint so far: missing his daily candy fix. After lunch, we take the elevator down to the main floor and locate the candy machine. As we walk through the public rooms, munching on our Mars bars, a couple walking the corridor arm in arm greet us and stop to talk.

"Bob had to come here; he couldn't manage at home," the woman tells us. "For me, it was my choice to join him. I've got a sickness of my own, but I could have stayed at home. We've been here for five years. It's a good place." After a bit more chat, they walk on and disappear around a corner. We wander into a large open space filled with groupings of sofas and wing chairs. Some other people are already seated. "Shall we join them?" I ask Ken with a look, and he nods his assent.

As soon as we're seated, Nigel, a larger-than-life Londoner with a booming voice, and Carol ("Hi, I'm Carol from Hamilton") smile and introduce themselves. It's a classic first-day-at-the-new-school scene. During the next fifteen or so minutes, as the four of us attempt a conversation, I get a glimpse of the wary kid Ken must have been back in junior high. When Nigel tells us at length about how lively the British are and what absolutely fabulous comics they make, Ken replies, "Yes, and they don't refrain from talking about it." At first, when Nigel doesn't respond, I think he hasn't heard Ken or is choosing to ignore the remark. But when he asks me for the third time in five minutes what part of London we lived in during our year there, the ha'penny finally drops: Nigel is probably in the early stages of Alzheimer's.

Still, the ice has been broken; it was a good start. I give

Ken a quick good-bye kiss and leave the three of them to chat. "I'll make sure he gets back to his room," Nigel's voice booms after me.

Later that afternoon, the phone rings. Ken is furious, and surprisingly articulate in his anger. "They've got me in prison here!" he shouts. "For some reason, they didn't take it well when I told them I was going home for a couple of hours. I explained that I would be back, but these people are impossible. They just don't want me to leave."

Neither of us had asked about whether Ken would be allowed to go out on his own, so I just reminded him that he had spoken well of the staff the day before.

"Yes, but they've gone bad," he insisted.

We spoke for a while. He was finally reassured when I reminded him that Corry had made plans to take him out for lunch on the morrow.

Wednesday: Today the phone hasn't stopped ringing. During the first call, Ken sounded fine. Then Corry called to report that the outing went well, and that he made no objection when it was time to return to the residence. However, the next time the phone goes off, it is with that ominous French ambulance ring reserved for the social worker.

May from the CCAC is not happy: "Mrs. Sobol, they just phoned to let me know your husband tried to leave! He has tried four times! And the last time, he actually succeeded! An attendant had to run after him and bring him back."

My good mood plummets.

"Do you know why he would do that?" she wants to know.

Recalling our chat with Nigel and Carol, I point out the most likely reason: this is a big change for Ken, the cat who has always walked by himself. Even back in college, he never took to dormitory life, and this is a dormitory with a permanently locked front door.

But maybe these are the wrong things to say. Maybe I'll get him branded as a troublemaker, which has happened from time to time in his life. I don't want some official to send out a directive banning him forever from staying at long-term residences. Probably my imagination is working overtime, but I plead his case.

"I think he'll be fine, May, once he gets used to the place," I say. "I've heard a lot of people take awhile to accustom themselves to the new routine. He can't be the first person in the place ever to try to leave, can he?"

When I add that I'll phone the staff and try to sort things out, she sounds relieved. However, when I place my call, it's now a different shift; the person who picked up can't answer my questions. In fact, the staff have can't find anybody who can talk about the incident or incidents first hand. Even Ken, when they put him on the line, no longer seems bothered about whatever it was that happened at the front door.

That evening, the phone rings again. "I hope you realize that you won't be able to come in tomorrow," Ken informs me. "They've got the whole place in lockdown. They're not allowing anyone in or out. And listen, they tell me you've decided I should stay several extra days—I'm not happy at all about that."

I explain that the plan hasn't altered; he is coming home Monday morning just as planned. "And John is visiting you tomorrow afternoon," I tell him. "He and Sophie are driving in from Ottawa right now. He'll be allowed in; I'm sure he will be able to handle it."

When the Ottawa contingent arrives, John listens to my account of the day's adventures and gives me a hug, saying, "Well, Mom, I'm glad he's there for awhile, being cared for properly. And I'm glad you're here, getting some rest. And now Sophie and I are here with you."

Three helpful, short sentences.

Thursday: While John visits Ken, I get to granddaughter-sit. How relaxing to spend some time with the newest genera-tion. Through some intuitive process, ten-year-old Sophie and six-year-old Ximena average out the four-year difference in their ages to pass the next two hours in a dizzying mov-able feast of improvised play—removing and putting into use the entire contents of the toy drawer, ferreting out my stock of pencils and markers, and arranging and rearranging the chairs, cushions, blankets, tea towels, dolls, and stuffed ani-mals in various permutations.

I don't get peace and quiet due to the continuous hum of girl-voiced playmaking. ("Let's get some more pillows, Ximena. We can fix up a house in the sunroom now!" "Okay, Sophie. Should I get the blankets, too?") But it's a form of peace, light years away from any of the problems associated with ageing. I settle in with a paper and coffee. The phone cooperates, too, by not ringing even once.

Over dinner, John reports he found Ken cheerful and eager to talk: "He went on about what an outstanding, impressive woman you are, Mom."

"Really?" I ask incredulously.

"Yes, really. Those were his words. Of course, on the other hand, he also talked about plans for making a getaway. He told me, 'Yeah, for sure I'll need Julian; he'll have to be there.'" Julian, our seventeen-year-old grandson, is six-foot-five (or six-ten if you include the Afro).

Friday, his fifth day into respite care, Ken looks up, startled, when I appear at the door to his room.

"They've made all these replicas of you," he announces. "Got them all over the place, but I knew they weren't real. I can tell you're the real you, and I'm so happy you're here now."

I want to hold back the hands on the clock to make the moment last, but Ken has already moved on.

"You know, I can't believe I fell for that old con job," he says. "The one where the guy asks you to hold something and uses sleight-of-hand to change it on you. Bait-and-switch. You know what I mean."

"Yes, I know."

"And the guy in the next room? He's got someone in there; they're screwing all the time—I can hear him through the door. They encourage that stuff here. It's a way of controlling you. One of the staff—it's so weird—we were in this small room and I was put in charge of the clothes, and she got naked and people misunderstood."

Help. I sign us out for a walk. Maybe the fresh air will drive out a few of Ken's delusions. At a nearby coffee shop, we find a table. He orders his favorite drink, a latte, but the instant he is finished, he pushes back his chair. "I'm ready to go back now."

In front of the residence, a bus is parked, its engine running. A young woman with papers in her hand detaches herself from the crowd of people standing around. She approaches and introduces herself to me, then glances up at Ken. "You know we would have been glad to have you join us, Ken. Maybe next time?"

He doesn't answer.

As the bus is pulling away, he says, "See how they turn every question around and try to put the problem on you?"

"What about the other clients? How do they seem?"

He frowns. "Oh, them. They're always smiling and saying, 'Hi, Ken.'"

Once we are in his room again, I pick up the photo collage that Jane and William have put together for him. Ken notices and takes it from me, studying it briefly. "That's what sustains me," he says, with the hint of a smile. "I love my whole family."

It was a mixed visit; I let it go. On my bus ride home this windblown spring day, my eye takes in the wisps of cloud flying across a cerulean sky, the reinvigorated grass, budding bushes, and tossing treetops, all an electric shade of green. Their brilliant color is such a psychedelic experience that a burst of happiness at being alive washes over me. I feel an intense pleasure in this world in all its third-millennium urban variety. If the Greeks were right and proportion is everything, my life this winter has been seriously out of whack: eighty percent caregiving, fifteen percent grandmothering, five percent "other." A few quiet days alone in the house have reshaped that order, made life a bit more balanced.

I don't think that Ken, if he were able to pay attention long enough to me to hear me describe it, would begrudge me this fleeting moment of nirvana.

Sunday: The day before Ken's due to arrive home, Jane and I go to visit him together. I've kept Jane informed of the week's ups and downs. As she drives, we are silent, wondering what we'll find today. In the room, she barely has a chance to give Ken a warm hug and say hello before he starts talking compulsively; it's soon clear to me that, overnight, he has moved from wariness to full-throttle paranoia. There is no point trying an outing, not even to the candy machine. Instead, Jane and I find two chairs and listen as he paces the room and rambles on about staff conspiracies, racial taunts, and all-night orgies.

Back in the car, we sit for a moment. "Bummer," Jane says.

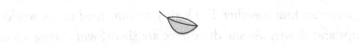

CHAPTER 14

Homecoming. As Ken and I walk down the street for a celebratory lunch, he takes my hand in his and says, "It feels wonderful to be back."

"Likewise," I reply, though I can't avoid the vaguely disloyal thought that his good mood is probably too good to last.

And it is. After lunch, when a friend phones to invite me out for coffee, Ken says he's fine with being left alone in the house for awhile. But he doesn't look fine. His hands are shaking more than usual. When I say I'll phone Laura back and cancel, he is obviously relieved.

"I'm just so scared," he whispers.

Only a year has passed since the two of us watched that short film in which British actress June Brown, looking straight into the camera, talked about her husband's LBD. While Ken is napping, I locate it on Google and watch again, paying close attention to one passage in particular:

[My husband] Robert became quite paranoid about seeing figures at the bottom of the garden. We had a kind of garden shed that was like a sort of summerhouse that he built himself. And he was always seeing people behind the windows, and they frightened him. I think that is the thing that is awful: the fear that [LBD] sufferers feel. Bob knew what was happening to him, and he hated it. He once said, "I never thought I'd go to the end like this," and then he [followed that] with, "I wish I were dead." It wasn't in a dramatic way. He just said, "I wish I were dead." It is a most *strange* disease, and I can't explain it to you, and I think it is worse than Alzheimer's because of this awareness of what you are going through.

It was one thing, before Ken had reached Robert's stage, to hear such an intense level of fear described. But observing it close up and personal is something else entirely. Still, the old pleasure in hearing his voice, in having him back here in our house, our house in the middle of the street, is still there.

I have missed him.

This next morning, the expression "safe as houses" just doesn't apply. Not for Ken, anyway—his fear is palpable. He is frantic to get away from the bad people lurking behind every door and around every corner. He takes a quick, furtive look before venturing into the hallway. Where can we go that he will feel safe? I wonder.

Corry comes by to take him on another diversionary outing, but when she brings him back, he refuses point blank to get out of car. It takes her several minutes to talk him into entering the house.

"There's no place like home." So says Dorothy, with girlish conviction. That oft-repeated line doesn't apply here. How awful it must feel to be afraid of your own familiar space, so terrified that you don't want to go inside, even with someone else there. On the evening news, I listen to reports about the millions who, in exile from home and homeland, are living year after year in "temporary" internment camps. Ken is like them, except he is in exile from not from home, but from himself.

And what a terrible, crushing loss that must be.

Serious illness sometimes has a way of bringing people together. Until a few days ago, when he asked me to dial her number for him, Ken and his younger sister had been out of touch for some time. Debbie was startled but pleased to hear his voice and wanted a chance to talk in person.

She and her husband, Fred, arrived yesterday from Boston. The atmosphere was strained at first, and the conversation mostly three-way, but I could tell that Ken was making an effort and that Debbie was clearly delighted to be back in touch, even at this late date. The reunion was as good as you could hope for, given the circumstances.

But the meeting only distracted Ken temporarily from his fears. After a bad night, he woke up this morning to a new crowd of his imaginary visitors.

"I am worried about you!" he says. "And nothing can be done about it! I'm ready to give up on you. You're too soft on these people."

I don't know which among his assortment of apparitions he means by "these people," but they have vanished by the time we sit down to dinner with Debbie and Fred. Ken is in good form during the meal, speaking frankly to Debbie about his symptoms, even trying out a few jokes about the unpredictable nature of his many hallucinations.

The following day, we turn tourist, heading down to Harbourfront with our guests. A stiff breeze coming off the lake buffets us as we stroll along the newly widened stretch of boardwalk. A visiting three-masted schooner and row of tour boats are doing a herky-jerky dance in their berths. After a quick tour through the colorful wall hangings and walrus sculptures in the Inuit Gallery, we drop into a waterfront café. Across the table from me, Ken, sitting with an Irish coffee in hand, looks weather-blown and almost carefree. I make a note to myself: there aren't any lurkers-behind-doors by the water; we should visit the lake again soon.

We're well into May, 2010 and Ken is still able to manage the bathroom by himself—for which we're probably both grateful—but most other daily living activities, including the computer, telephone, TV remote, radio, food prep, medication, shopping, and doctor's appointments, now require supervision. Zippers and buttons are the newest challenge; on bad days, he has trouble figuring out which foot goes into which pant leg.

He remains fussy about his appearance. No sooner was

he dressed this morning than I heard drawers being opened and closed. "I don't like the blue t-shirt anymore. Where's that black one, the one with 'Writer's Guild' on the pocket?" he asks. I look around. The bedroom furniture is draped with items worn briefly and then airily discarded. Clumps of unmatched socks huddle together in corners; his underwear drawer, full only a couple of days ago, is now empty. Do clothes act as a protective layer between Ken and the increasingly scary outside world?

Because the washing machine in the basement is reached via a trap door and steep flight of stairs, I am delighted by a morning phone call from the CCAC offering us three hours per week of help. The PCW (personal care worker) assigned to us is available to begin whenever I'd like, and at no charge. For me, the news is as welcome as a lottery win.

Only a couple of days later, Doti, beautifully dreadlocked and single-mindedly efficient, arrives for her first day as Ken's personal care worker. It's our first experience with the service, which apparently includes assistance with everything from laundry and personal care to tidying the client's room and providing informal counseling. Doti is something like a free-lance nanny and maid-of-all-work, but better paid and with a better, well-deserved status.

In no time at all, our female Jeeves has Ken showered, shampooed, and dressed in clean clothes. She deals just as quickly with our disreputable fridge, tossing out leftovers and unidentifiable, soggy vegetables without a moment's hesitation, leaving the interior cleaner than it has been since it left the factory.

"Any other jobs that need doing?" she asks.

I like this woman.

I leave her to tidy the bedroom and go into the living room. Seated in his favorite chair, where Doti has deposited him, Ken looks so sparkling, glowing, squeaky clean that he might be a younger version of himself. The fact that our PCW is young, attractive, and has a good sense of humor might be contributing to his easy acceptance of to what could be seen as a humiliating experience.

May 18: Corry's husband, Greg, has invited Ken to watch the basketball game at their place. I watch with them for a few minutes and then, feeling like one of the Vichy sympathizers in the film *Casablanca*, say I'm going out for a walk when the truth is I've arranged a rendezvous with my other kids at a bar around the corner. The sense of betrayal that haunts dementia caregivers is very present as I pull the door shut behind me. Though I long ago gave up on sleeping through the night and have dropped pleasurable activities like tai chi and art class because Ken can't be left alone (and he strongly resists the suggestion of having a stranger keep him company), it never seems to be enough.

This year's spring has been one small, downward lurch after another: Ken's communication struggles, the fall in the laneway, the second house obsession, and the heightened level of fear about every aspect of life. Plus, there are worsening physical problems, such as his persistent cough. I know a major event of some kind is inevitable, though the doctors can't predict whether it would be weeks or months away.

In the bar, the four of us crowd into a booth. Almost three years have passed since the Father's Day get-together when we sat in stunned silence, trying to absorb the fact that our husband/father needed help. We were neurological neophytes at that point: disbelieving, unprepared, and unfamiliar with dementia. Things are radically different now; during those three years, our family has gained the equivalent of a group PhD in LBD and its disorienting effects on the personality—Ken's unpredictable jumps and dips in cognition, the strange remarks, the memory lapses.

Tonight the question at hand is whether or not I should phone the CCAC and ask for Ken to be put on the list for crisis care, knowing we would have to accept whatever bed was available, at whatever location. It is a true dilemma, so we take a vote. Corry and Jane vote to act right away; John and I opt to wait a little longer in the hope we get lucky with a place on our list of top choices. But, numbers aside, we are united in wishing there were a third alternative—like news of some wonderfully innovative residence opening in the neighborhood, a windfall inheritance from some unknown relative so that I could buy a house and hire round-the-clock help, or a miracle cure.

The four co-conspirators walk back in gloomy silence to make small talk with Ken and Greg about who won the game and how many baskets the star forward scored.

A few days after the secret meeting, Ken and I are back at our warm-weather station on the front porch. It's lovely to be able to sit outside again. As we watch the passing parade of dog walkers and stroller pushers, he suddenly breaks the silence: "Look at all these people going by, all the people sitting on their porches. Just look at them!"

His urgent tone catches my attention.

"Don't you realize how alarming this is?" he continues, turning to look at me. "Haven't you noticed how they can put their thoughts into your mind? It's you I'm worried about—the danger. One of them could easily pick something up and smash you over the head. Do you understand?"

I start to say he doesn't have to worry about me, that I can take care of myself, but he interrupts.

"And those theater people..." he says. "You're one of them, you know."

"I am?" I ask cautiously. This was news to me.

"Yes, haven't you even noticed that elaborate costume you're wearing?"

The question is asked with such total conviction that I find myself glancing down to check. (I am still wearing the capris and top I put on earlier that morning.)

"We'll have to get rid of those theater people," Ken repeats. "They're trouble-makers."

But if I am one of them, one of the imaginary players who have apparently followed him home from his short-term stay, am I, too, a troublemaker? I didn't ask the question out loud.

In the early days of Ken's hallucinations, as we lay in bed at four in the morning discussing the latest visions, I used to wonder why I didn't just run out the door. The answer I always gave myself was that that's what people do when there's no other choice.

The truth is that, through years of watching him deal night after night with the changing roster of creatures, I have never felt afraid—discomfited, saddened, worried, overwhelmed, sleep-deprived, sure, but never afraid. Ken has expressed his own worries on the subject occasionally, though—like the time we watched a documentary that showed an Alzheimer's patient pinching and pulling hair as his wife got him ready for bed. The scene was so troubling that someone could be heard off-screen trying to intervene.

"I can be rather unpleasant at times," Ken had reminded me when the film ended.

Today's disjointed accusatory conversation has made me uncomfortable. I know it's not unusual for dementia patients to talk in alarming ways; I also know the overwhelming majority don't become violent beyond the occasional push or pinch. But still. I am starting to not like the thought of being alone with him when he's roaming the house at three a.m. and I'm sound asleep.

I'm glad John is here now for a few days; I decide that once he leaves, I will tell our daughters not to be surprised if they get a phone call from me asking for company at night.

CHAPTER 15

In my dream, a babble of sound is coming from our front vestibule. A small boy keeps asking, "What's the matter with the man, Dad?"

Another voice, which seems familiar says, "Where's Julie? Somebody get her."

Here I am. Don't you see me? I open my eyes, but the noise continues. It wasn't a dream. John must already have left for his business meeting. What was going on?

Slipping into my robe, I hurry to the front door to find Ken barefoot, wearing his old blue nightshirt with a quilt from our country auction days draped over one arm. He is surrounded by a group of people who seem to have emerged from the set of a sitcom. Two paramedics in full belted and looped regalia are speaking earnestly with a couple of men I've never seen before in my life. A couple of neighbors stand behind them, just watching. The little boy is Lucas, our landlord's son. Some other faces seem vaguely familiar from walks around the neighborhood.

One of the strangers steps up. "He told me he was looking for medical help." The others turn and stare at me; they seem to be demanding action, but what is the protocol? I invite the two medics, one of whom has Ken by the hand, to come inside. As I pull the door firmly shut behind them, I hear the crowd disperse, talking among themselves as they return to their own lives.

Ken falls into a chair without speaking. The medics explain that a stranger noticed him wandering around and stopped to ask him if he needed help. A second man noticed the Alzheimer's Society medic alert bracelet on Ken's wrist and phoned the police. The medics ask the usual questions—when did the illness start, has he ever done this before, what medications does he take, what are the dosages—and then, after giving him a quick once-over, hurry on out to confront their next emergency.

How long had he been out there? I wondered. Two minutes? Two hours? I hadn't thought to ask the names of his rescuers, so I wouldn't be able to thank them. Ken, who by now is looking more alert, tries to fill me in. "Those two men that brought me home? I've noticed them before. They've been watching the house for days. That's the only reason they spoke to me. They're planning a break-in. We have to be careful."

For once, I remember to obey the "do not reality-orient" rule and redirect the conversation. Ken's previous "lost" moments were just a matter of momentary disorientation.

During the bank episode he had the good sense to look at the cards in his wallet and remember that, yes, he was indeed Ken Sobol. This was different. He went out in his nightshirt, for starters. And if he had wanted to check his wallet, he couldn't have; he'd left it at home along with his keys, glasses, and shoes.

He might have wandered miles away if no one had been curious about the barefoot Diogenes carrying not a lantern but a patchwork quilt. Okay, this was Toronto—that wouldn't have happened. But he could have walked in front of a truck, or...or anything could have happened.

I phone the social worker associated with Ken's geriatrician to ask her advice. "Julie," she says, "this is what you have to do. You have to go to the hardware store and buy a small slide bolt for your front door. It works every time—keeps them from wandering out in the middle of the night. If you put it up high, he won't even notice."

I tell her that I'll give her suggestion a try, and since I have her on the line anyway, I raise my concern about the increased aggression. "I wouldn't worry yet," she reassures me. "These things he's saying are part of his attempt to make sense of the world while his mind gradually disintegrates."

As I am about to hang up, she adds, "If he ever starts talking about killing, though, that's something else. Then it's time for action."

The following day, William comes by and installs the slide bolt. It will prove useful in the future.

I can locate lost keys if I look long enough, but where do I look for a lost house, a house that doesn't exist in time and space? Do I try the yellow pages? Google "non-architects"? I have read of one dementia patient whose version of the doubling phenomenon involved the house where he grew up, a real structure in a faraway city. "If I knew where this other house of yours was," I say to Ken, "if it were in Cleveland, or Montreal, or wherever, I'd go looking with you. Really. But I don't know."

All day I watch him struggle with this existential quandary. When dusk arrives, and the street light in front of the house flickers on, he is still fretting. I can't watch silently anymore. As we descend the front steps, I wonder what is going to happen when he doesn't find what he's looking for.

At the sidewalk, Ken hesitates before taking a left. We stroll in silence as far as the small corner park where, during the day, our youngest grandchildren are often among the crowd swinging across the monkey bars or improving their hole-digging skills in the sandbox. At this hour, the place is deserted except for the usual huddle of teenagers at one of the picnic tables. As we walk past them, one boy who might be all of fifteen is telling his friends, "When I was younger, I used to really like…" But noticing us, he immediately lowers his voice, and I don't get to find out which girl or rock band or questionable substance he really liked so long ago.

Ken stops at the edge of the empty wading pool, evidently unsure about how to proceed. I stand a few feet away. I can't think of any words that would help prompt him toward a next step. Time passes. *They also serve who only stand and wait*, I think, remembering Milton's famous words. *But for how long?* I turn and start, very slowly, to leave the park.

Ken calls after me, "I don't even want to walk with you! I'm very angry!"

Apparently, it was my fault the house wasn't waiting for him under the dark trees. I find it difficult, even now, to express why this moment, for me, was the lowest point so far in our Lewy Body journey. Perhaps it was simply that over the years we had helped each other through so many daily challenges; before his illness there always was—as in any healthy relationship—a rough equality in the demands we placed on each other. The ratio at any given moment didn't have to be fifty-fifty because you knew, when the other person seemed over-demanding, that you had occasionally demanded more than your share of the pie, too.

But it is harder now, when Ken needs so much attention, so much sympathy, to accept that he has (as far as I can tell) absolutely zero sense of my parallel ordeal. Instead of realizing that I am trying to help him find his way through his trials, he views me as the cause of them. I know he is sick, but the lack of balance in our relationship is against all logic, all the laws of human life, and just so *strange*.

At times like this, the disconnect between professionals and family caregivers becomes not a gap but a canyon. How many of the doctors and psychologists who write books and articles about dementia, and who advocate wonderfully creative ways of dealing with each new symptom, are working on a 24/7/365 basis? In real life, away from the classroom or the lab, you can reach the point where you are too immersed in the details of the situation to come up with one more simple-yet-brilliant practical solution. Even Sherlock Holmes couldn't have solved the case of "The House that Wasn't There in the Night."

When I reach our front walk, Ken trailing behind me, I don't want to go in the house—not while he is in this angry mood. I stay out on the porch for a long time. He comes and peers at me from the door.

The next morning, Ken wants to try another search. I remind him that Carol and David Bady, old friends who have driven up from New York to see him, are coming for lunch. He stares at me briefly and asks when we will "get all this [i.e., the double house] sorted out." The belligerence level is high enough to prompt me to phone the Badys and ask for help. David says they'll be right over.

Our friendship with these two people has lasted half a century; Carol and I were dorm mates before I had even met Ken. David served as an usher at our wedding, and it was he who, taking us born-and-bred Midwesterners under his Brooklyn-born, Columbia-educated wing, shepherded us to the Judson Church forum that inspired Ken's first *Village Voice* piece. We have watched each other's children grow up and start families of their own; shared similar musical tastes, swapped family stories, and tolerated each other's political rants.

On their arrival, Ken greets Carol and David with more warmth than he has shown to anyone for a long time. Over a good lunch and a bottle of wine, Ken and I forget about phantom houses and Lewy Bodies as the four of us are transformed into a near version of our twenty-something selves during our White Horse Tavern days. Ken even tolerates David's persuasive argument for thinking more realistically about the eventual—or perhaps near—prospect of long-term care.

While Ken is napping, Corry drops by to say hello to our friends. As we sit around catching up, Ken suddenly appears in the doorway, a baseball bat raised high above his head (the one he keeps in the bedroom against potential burglars). He looks ready to hit someone. Is he joking or not? David gets up, gently removes the bat, and someone puts it out of sight. For the next few minutes, everybody tries to be in the moment as they search for the right words to say or not say, until Ken, in the usual pattern, comes out of his daze and looks around.

"I think I could eat something," he says. We choose a nearby place with a quiet patio; Greg joins us, too. While five people study their menus and banter with the waiter in the warmth of the late afternoon sun, the sixth person is barely a presence, off somewhere on his own planet.

Unfortunately, when Carol and David left, they took the good times with them. Ken is now refusing to stay in the house, though he can't say where he would like to go. The haughty tone has returned. He tells me, after thinking it over, "I want to talk to our children. Take me to one of their houses, please."

We head out to the garage. Since Jane is already at work at this hour, it is Corry who gets to look startled when she opens her door at nine a.m. to find her parents standing outside like a pair of discomfited religious recruiters. I've never needed Corry's presence of mind more than I do now, and she doesn't let me down.

One glance at Ken tells her something is up. She hurries us inside and settles him down with the paper and a cup of coffee. This appears to be a safe house for Ken. When Teddy, their frisky poodle, decides the visitor needs company and bounds into his lap, Ken looks down, scratches him between the ears, and murmurs, "How're you doing, Teddy?"

Corry and I climb the stairs to their home office. After the events of the last five days, there is no need for discussion; I'd already dropped my last qualms about crisis care. I knew it might take the CCAC as long as two or three weeks to find a bed, so we had to act quickly. Corry phones the CCAC while I search online for more residences to flesh out the short list I had given them earlier.

Wrapping up her conversation, Corry puts down the phone. "Mom, there's something I have to tell you," she says. I look up. *What now?* "John had an emergency operation on his gall bladder last night. He'd been having pain for a few days, but he and Annie, thought it was just indigestion." Seeing the worry in my face, she quickly adds, "He's fine now, absolutely fine. But we didn't want to tell you until we knew it was okay. You've had enough on your mind."

She's right about that.

Only after Annie assures me over the phone that John is doing fine do I feel calm enough to tell Ken. He would likely sense something was wrong, anyway, and maybe having someone else to worry about might help take him out of himself. Sure enough, it does. He takes the news calmly, or as calmly as I did. He repeats over and over, "Just as long as he's fine now."

However, he has noticed our long absence upstairs and

is curious about all of the phone calls. Corry plunges in. "Dad, we know you don't want to go back to Wellesley. We're looking at some other residences on the list." That was true enough as far as the phone calls went. I would never send him back there, though Wellesley wasn't at fault—I had no complaints about their level of care. But he didn't feel that way, and right now I want to avoid mentioning anything that might touch off a new bout of fear.

Corry and I are clearing up the lunch dishes when Ken wanders into the kitchen. "Could you both come and sit down, please," he requests. "There's something I think we have to get clear; I want to speak to you both about Dolma."

Ever since John left, I've had someone sleeping on the sofa every night. Dolma, a recently arrived Tibetan refugee who exudes an unearthly calm, is one of the personal care workers who has filled in when family wasn't available. On her first night with us, she had managed so well that I didn't hear a thing until she woke me at six a.m. "Three times he tried to leave, Julie," she had told me the next morning. "He said he wanted to go out to look for medical help. But that little slide bolt was a good idea. The door didn't open but he didn't seem to notice the lock. I talked to him for a while, and before he went back to bed he told me he trusted me."

Making anyone's acquaintance for the first time when they show up at 10 p.m. for an eight-hour job shift is a good test of your hospitality skills. You have to make the worker feel welcome (the arrangement is as strange for them as it is for you), then provide a coherent summary of the illness, and make sure he or she knows the layout (where the bathroom is, where the extra blankets are kept). I have welcomed these women with open arms. I need their help and I regard them as friends. It is different for Ken—I know that. For him, they are one more reminder of his rapidly vanishing privacy and sense of self-respect. But with the workers here, I could get eight hours of sleep and be in better shape for the next day.

After Dolma's second night with us, Ken came to me and, almost like a spoken word poet, recited:

"This is how my day begins:

I waken, get up, find a woman from Tibet in my living room.

This woman bars my path whichever way I turn.

Why do we need her,

this woman from Tibet?

Where does she come from?

She comes up from underground to get in my way."

In light of his "performance" that day, I can't say his request for a talk about Dolma comes as a surprise.

"I like Dolma," he begins, as Corry joins me on the sofa. "Really, she's all right. But there are problems. For one thing, you've given her too many hours. I absolutely do not want her to stay more than nine. Nine is the maximum."

I tell him that's fine. (A skewed perception of time is another LBD symptom.)

"Good. Next, she is to leave me alone *unless I ask for help*—is that clear? I don't want people to keep asking me if I'm alright. I don't like it."

I assure him that I will speak to Dolma, that she will be cooperative. But the morning is moving on. Corry, who is homeschooling Elliot, her youngest, glances at the clock. I remind Ken that we are keeping them from their work. He gets up willingly.

Back home again, the change in his demeanor is striking. The house obsession has disappeared for now, and he seems so much more comfortable with me and with himself that the occasional delusional—but not hostile—remark dropped into the conversation isn't bothersome. Apparently, we have for some unknown reason acquired a half-ton truck.

"What do you want to do with that truck, anyway?" Ken asks.

"Sell it?"

"Okay, we'll do that," he says with an easy shrug.

Maybe the news of John's operation has grounded him emotionally, maybe he was pleased about his successful stand on the Dolma issue, or maybe he just needed an extra dose of TLC. When you're in distress, you crave kindness as much as you do an analgesic.

CHAPTER 16

The next morning when the crisis came, it caught me off guard. Denial had crept in just as I was congratulating myself for doing such a good job of avoiding it. Everything was fine when Ken came into my room around three a.m. to tell me which filly was going to win the next race. We spoke briefly, he returned to bed, and I fell asleep...

Until about five a.m.

I got up to investigate a noise and found him standing in the hall near the bathroom. His eyes were open and he was conscious, but he couldn't manage his legs and he was unable to talk except for a couple of mumbled words. I felt his forehead; it was clammy, but this didn't look like a heart attack; he wasn't in pain, wasn't clutching his chest or falling over. Was this what catatonia looked like? He seemed to want the bathroom. I helped him onto the toilet, but nothing much happened. However, when I lifted him off, I found blood on the seat and more blood in the bowl.

I wasn't thinking all that clearly, and it seemed important to get him cleaned up before our next move. *One step at a time.* Somehow, I got him into the shower and positioned him under the spray. It was hard to manipulate the controls while keeping a good hold on him, but he didn't comment on the rush of tepid water.

Corry, on sofa duty that night, was awakened by the sound of our crashing around in the shower. She stood at the door briefly, yawning and rubbing her eyes, then quickly grabbed a towel to help me dry him and pull the stretchy fabric of a nightshirt over his damp, uncooperative bulk. Corry held him up while I hurried away to grab a kitchen chair. Our little group performed a Three Stooges shuffle in the narrow hallway as we tried to get him to bend his knees enough to be lowered into position. Bursts of nervous laughter escaped from Corry and me at the unlikely, awkward strangeness of this pre-dawn scene. Ken appeared to be wide awake, but was oblivious.

I phoned 911 and within minutes the doorbell rang. Luckily, Isaac and Greg, the medics who took care of Ken when he fell in the laneway, responded to the call. They remembered the incident and handled him gently. There was a quick debate once we were in the ambulance about which hospital to head for. After consulting their computer, they and decided to opt for Toronto Western because it was having a relatively light night. (A good choice, as it turned out; though I didn't know at the time, Western is known for its advanced work in neurological research.)

Our experience with Ontario hospitals had been consistently good, but I took to this one as soon as we were through the ER doors. A doctor from the surgical team ordered blood tests and quickly directed a nurse to have Ken moved into a cubicle with a bed. Once we were resettled, a gastroenterologist arrived to take a lengthy medical history. By that point, the morning had advanced and I hadn't eaten so much as a slice of toast. I had answered many repeats of the same questions—understandable 'given the different medical people and Ken's confusing array of symptoms—but suddenly there was just one question too many. The doctor, noticing my tears, stopped in mid-sentence.

"Take as much time as you need, Mrs. Sobol," he told me. We found two chairs. He said, "We're thinking of doing a colonoscopy. How do you feel about that?"

I explained that, in his current state, Ken would almost certainly need to be anaesthetized for such an invasive procedure and that it was the anesthetic used in the TURP procedure that had triggered his first hallucinations. And that was when he was in better shape, both physically and cognitively. I didn't like to think about how it would it affect him now. "I'm not sure what purpose the test would serve, anyway." I added. "If they found cancer, he couldn't handle an operation, much less the radiation treatments." The doctor didn't say so, but I got the feeling was thinking the same thing. In the end, I agreed to a sigmoidoscopy, a mini version of the longer test. He thanked me for my help and left to make arrangements to have Ken admitted to the surgery ward.

The next morning, I woke at five a.m. after a heavy sleep and was at the hospital by eight. Ken's sixth-floor room looked out over a roof covered with scaffolding, but he didn't care about the view—still out of it this morning, no real conversation. A plastic tube emerged from under his blanket, running down to a bottle filled with reddish liquid.

I had trouble finding anyone on the busy surgical ward who could give me a prognosis or tell me how long he would be staying. Two of the nurses stopped by to introduce themselves, but were quickly called away to respond to buzzers, tend the patients, and maneuver gurneys carrying groggy-looking post-op patients back to their rooms.

Around noon, an attendant arrived to take Ken downstairs for his sigmoidoscopy. I went home to let in our once-a-week housekeeper. By now, I was convinced there was something gravely wrong with him, and Silvana's concerned inquiry about how Mr. Sobol was doing brought on another flood of tears. But when the phone rang, it was good news. "We found no major problems, Mrs. Sobol," a doctor told me. "The blood in his urine is probably just from inserting the catheter—that happens sometimes. Not to worry, your husband will be able to return home today."

A flood of doubt immediately tempered my brief rush of euphoria. I'd done a fair bit of home nursing in my time, but Grandma Macfie had remained an active participant in her own care; she made her needs known, participated in medical decisions, functioned as a valued member of the family;

Ken, in contrast, was in a near-crisis state even before yesterday's early-morning attack. He would be coming home incontinent, unable to feed himself (unable to manage food at all without the major worry of choking), and unable to walk without help. He was not communicating clearly about pain, either. How long would I be able to maintain the level of care that he needed? (That question would be answered for me within thirty-six hours.)

When Corry brought Ken home in the ambulance, she was worried too. "I tried to argue with them, Mom," she said. "No one would listen. All the way home, Dad was sure the ambulance was taking him to jail." She smiled briefly to herself, shook her head, and then explained, "He wouldn't believe me when I kept telling him he was going home. You should have heard him when we turned onto your street. He could see a bit out the little window, and as we pulled up in front of the house, he stopped rambling and said, very clearly, 'Well, I'll be damned!' You had to laugh."

By late afternoon, Jane, William, and Greg had joined us. Everyone got to work making lists, clearing shelves, compiling a complicated schedule of who could help at what times. People made forays to the drugstore and returned with loaded bags. Corry took a box of adult diapers from one of the bags and examined the chart on the side. "They're the wrong size," she said. Greg offered to go back and exchange them for larger ones.

By the time the younger generation left, the place resembled a real sickroom. Neatly arranged boxes of tissues, stacks of diapers, and bottles of lotion and antiseptic covered every free surface. And when Marie-Cruz, tonight's PCW, arrived at ten, she somehow managed to get across to Ken that constantly tugging on the catheter was not a wise move. A small balloon keeps the tube in place inside the bladder, she explained, and if he pulled that out he would find the experience very painful indeed.

The clock read 6:30 a.m. when I awoke. I found Jane in Ken's bedroom, chatting in Spanish with Marie-Cruz. Jane had stopped by en route to work to check on how things were going. I watched as they worked at the simple job of getting Ken washed and changed; since he was a dead weight this involved lots of lifting and tugging for the two of them, but they managed.

Around ten, a visiting nurse arrived. "I'm Vladislov," he told us. "But don't worry about getting the name right—no one does." He took in our careful arrangements with one brief professional glance. His comment? "You people won't be able to manage this." Yes, we had got the right size of diaper, he acknowledged, and that was good, but they were the wrong model. "The side-opening ones are better in this situation." I hadn't even known there were side-opening diapers. After checking the catheter and measuring Ken's urine output, Vladislov wished us luck and left us to get on with our work as best we could.

Nursing a dementia patient, it turns out, is complicated. Ken had so many different symptoms to deal with. No one had said a word yet about his sudden loss of mobility. Just three days ago, he had negotiated the six-block walk from the restaurant with David at his side. I phoned Ken's physical therapist to ask his opinion about trying a few steps. Mario mulled it over. He thought it was worth a try but advised us to use caution. With one of us holding Ken firmly on each side, we carefully got him standing. His feet immediately flopped out from under him, and he crumpled.

Not encouraging. We decide to forget about mobility for now.

After lunch, when I brought him some juice, he looked up at me and, for the first time since returning home, seemed to take in the scene. Handing me the emptied glass, he said calmly, "I love you, you know." Then, in another of those formal moods that blend self-parody and real gravity, he said, "Now I want to talk to my children." I called in Jane and Corry, who joined him on the big bed and waited expectantly.

"I'm going to die soon, both of us are," he told them. Normally I wouldn't be wild about being tossed casually into this conversation, but it was good to hear him talking in full sentences again. Even with his mind in this disordered state, he was trying his best to come to terms with the situation, and he wanted to help us do the same.

"After I'm gone," he continued, "I don't want all you people to stick around here. Just get right back to what you're doing."

It was hard to know what to say to this.

"Do you understand?" he asked them. They both nodded. "Good."

He turned to me and said, "Now, please go and get the men."

I started to explain that John was in Ottawa and William and Greg had gone home, but his eyes were already closing. The brief speech had used up his small store of energy.

The rest of the day passed somehow. Despite Vladislov's gloomy prediction, we had made it through a second day.

Last night when the personal care worker didn't show up at ten, Corry insisted on waiting up with me and I didn't argue. When I woke this morning I found her on the sofa; it turned out the worker had never shown up, had not even phoned. I was concerned. Tomorrow was Monday and everyone had other responsibilities to return to. It was becoming clear that to care properly for someone who is both bedridden and suffering from advanced dementia, you need round-the-clock help—preferably from two dependable and physically strong people, at least one of whom is experienced in specialized nursing.

In the morning light, I rethought Vladislov's prophecy and made a few calls. The person who answered at one agency said they had an experienced woman who just moved here from North Bay; Lori was her name and she could start that afternoon. Was I interested?

I hired Lori for twenty-four hours, to begin this afternoon at five p.m. *From here on,* I told myself, *we'll take it one day at a time.*

By five-thirty p.m., everything was under control. Ken was in bed asleep. Lori and I were in the kitchen preparing supper. As I peeled potatoes and she assembled salad, I listened to her chat about her kids, her new apartment, the special courses she had taken in dementia care. After adding the dressing, she set the salad on the table. "I'll just go check on Ken," she said. A moment later, I was startled to hear a shout.

"Julie, come here! Come right away! He's out of bed and he's pulled out his catheter. He's bleeding…he's holding my wrists! Hurry, I need you right now!"

I rushed down the hall to see Ken and Lori facing each other like a pair of Greco-Roman wrestlers, rocking back and forth, the catheter dangling loose, blood everywhere. Lori, very professionally and calmly, repeated over and over, "Don't hurt me, Ken. I won't hurt you. I'm here to help you. Don't hurt me, please. Don't twist my wrists. I don't want to harm you."

He looked up when I entered the room but didn't speak. As they continued to arm wrestle, I reached for the phone and, within minutes, we were rushed back to the ER and then whisked up to the same sixth-floor room Ken had left just two days ago.

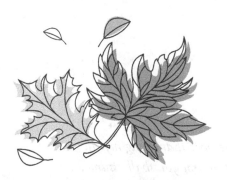

Part III

Crisis Care

I celebrate my self and sing myself,
And what I assume you shall assume...
  —Walt Whitman, *Leaves of Grass*

The mind is enough.
  —Gwen Furmark, friend

CHAPTER 17

When Gwen Furmark and I were young mothers living in Brooklyn, we used to see a lot of each other. However, since our move to Canada, we had lost touch. It was as if the earth had swallowed her up; she and Roy weren't in the city phone book anymore, and no one seemed to know where they had gone—until a call in 1988 from a mutual friend. She had run into someone who knew one of Gwen's relatives, and the news wasn't good. A sudden, massive brain infection had left Gwen completely paralyzed, unable even to speak. No wonder the long silence.

When I told Ken, we made a mutual vow to never, ever, to complain again about our own lot. A promise not kept, of course, but I did act quickly on my decision to write Gwen. I didn't know if I would hear back—Roy must have his hands full. However, within a couple of weeks, I had received an envelope addressed by Roy. The letter inside had been typed by Gwen, using a mouthstick and electric typewriter. In it she complained about what ageing and years in a wheelchair had done to her muscle tone, especially her "thunder thighs."

The last time I saw her, Gwen was no longer working professionally as a dancer, but was still taking classes. I couldn't picture that vibrant athlete's body in a wheelchair. My own regret at going from size eight to fourteen during that period seemed embarrassingly trivial in comparison. *Was* trivial. Mostly, though, during what would turn out to be a long correspondence, Gwen didn't dwell on her illness. "How strong the human body is," she wrote once. "We can withstand so much. Keeping the brain intact is most important…family and friends caring about each other…Yessir, that's what it's all about…Keep busy, stay active. It'll keep you young."

Coming from anyone else, these would have been Hallmark truisms; from Gwen Furmark, they acquired fresh relevance.

Later, in the mid-nineties, Roy phoned to say he was coming to Toronto on business and was toying with the idea of bringing Gwen—that is, if we could keep her company while he attended a meeting. Two weeks later, we met them in their hotel lobby. As we walked in, I spotted Roy leaning casually against the counter, Gwen seated not far away and staring intently in our direction. When I got closer, I found that despite the admittedly shrunken body and stiffly crossed arms, she looked as chic as ever in her ski sweater and stylish jeans. Her eyes were bright and behind them you could sense the dammed-up words wanting to cascade out.

Roy did most of the talking over lunch. We learned that

the family had gone through a series of less-than-perfect helpers until one day he announced to Gwen that he, with the help of their two teenage boys, would take on the job, and they had done just that ever since. (I had to revise my view of Roy as a jet-setting, hard-driven financial manager.) After hundreds of hours with a speech therapist, Gwen had regained some ability to talk. "Though it takes some people awhile to understand her," he cautioned.

When Roy headed off for his meeting, we took the elevator up to their room, Ken pushing Gwen in her chair. For the next several hours, the three of us sat together in that anonymous-looking space, and while the light slowly faded outside the large window, we worked at the arduous task of communicating. Ken did better than I did at catching on to Gwen's throaty vowels and muffled consonants, but even so it was slow going. Each phrase, sometimes each individual syllable, had to be repeated more than once. But no one was waiting for us downstairs—we could take all the time in the world.

I asked Gwen what she did with her time. Keeping busy wasn't a problem, she explained, not for either of them. Roy had his hands full running the house and tending to her needs. She had learned to paint a few years back, using her mouthstick, and she liked doing that. She watched TV— sitcoms, talk shows, and political debates; she thought a lot about old times and old friends and sometimes wrote to the latter; and she enjoyed sitting on the deck of their Vermont mountain home to watch the seasons change. "I see lots of... birds," she said. "Some...times a deer...stands...looking at me."

As I pictured the scene she described, a poem—as often happens—popped unbidden into my head. This time it was Robert Frost's "Two Look at Two," the one in which a young couple is climbing a wooded trail when they turn a corner and come face-to-face with a doe. The two humans and the woods creature stand silently watching each other for several moments before the human pair turn to go. Just then, there's a rustling of branches and an enormous stag emerges from the brush to stand beside his mate. The cross-species encounter comes full circle.

Gwen misread my momentary silence; she thought I needed reassuring about her condition. She declared, with conviction, "It's not a problem. The mind is enough."

The mind is enough. Since that afternoon in the hotel room, I've thought often about Gwen's remark. Her mind was as sharp as ever, perhaps sharper because of the challenges that fate had put her through, and she had learned to remain involved despite her body letting her down. But the reverse wasn't true, was it? What good was a strong body without the mind? Ken could still walk and talk (or had been able to before the crisis), but his mind...

I keep wondering how long, once the brain starts undergoing a catastrophic physical assault, do you retain a sense of self? And what is "self," anyway? Are there different levels of consciousness, of self-awareness, at different points in our lives? Can dementia patients hold on to a portion of their pre-dementia core right to the end? If they can, what is the glue that holds the self together? Or, if they can't, then at what point in the slow dance of this weird, relentless disease do they begin to lose that essential core?

You can get lost in this subject. In the hopes of better understanding what was happening to Ken, I had been reading everything I came across that touched on selfhood, but everyone had a slightly different answer. For linguist and psychologist Michael Corvallis, the mark of human selfhood is the ability to embed a phrase about the past in one about the present ("Pierre, the biologist who used to work at the Rockefeller Institute, now wants to become a rock musician.") Corvallis' term for this uniquely human ability is the "recursive mind." Neuroscientist Antonio Damasio, however, prefers the term "autobiographical self" to describe the way we use language, reasoning, and memory to achieve long-term plans; it's that ability, he believes, that leads to the flexibility and creativity which are key to the development of human society. Icelandic philosopher Kristjan Kristjansson uses simple words such as *commitments*, *hopes*, and *ideals* in his discussion of self as a person's central characteristics.

What ties all these outlooks together is a shared emphasis on memory and speech. Ken was struggling with both of these. Without memory you can't make sense of your overall life experience; without words you can't explain your self to others. Earlier this winter, after he reacted to a clever bit of repartee on some television show, I had told him, "It's so good to hear you laughing."

"Yeah," he had replied. "The dumb guy laughs." *So sad.*

Psychologist and author Tom Kitwood, in the early days of his career, had also asked questions about selfhood. As he got to know his dementia patients better, Kitwood was increasingly bothered by the way they were treated in hospitals—or, rather, not treated (he uses the phrase, "unattended dementia").

Kitwood tried to picture what the internal life of a dementia patient might be like:

> You are in a swirling fog and in half-darkness. You are wandering around in a place that seems vaguely familiar, and yet you do not know where you are; you cannot make out whether it is summer or winter, day or night. At times the fog clears a little, and you can see a few objects really clearly; but as soon as you start to get your bearings, you are overpowered by a kind of dullness and stupidity; your knowledge slips away, and again you are utterly confused. While you are stumbling in the fog you have an impression of people rushing past you, chattering like baboons. They seem to be so energetic and purposeful, but their business is incomprehensible…. Sometimes you catch sight of a familiar face; but as you move toward the face it vanishes, or turns into a demon. You feel desperately lost, alone, bewildered, frightened…
> But worst of all, it wasn't always like this.

Lost, alone, bewildered, frightened. That most be how Ken was feeling as he grew steadily worse.

I thought back to the class where he and I had first met, the one with the high-brow title of "Introspection and Observation: Philosophical Aspects of Psychoanalysis." At the opening of each session, one of the two professors would chalk a few words on the board, then turn to face us and politely request us to "discuss." During one class, Mr. Buck picked up the chalk. "The Law of Interchangeability of Pronouns," he wrote, "leads us to think it makes sense to suppose Jones can do something logically but not empirically." Then the stinger: "How do we know what emotions other people are feeling?"

This query sounded simple enough—that is, until you tried to answer it. A couple of the braver students stumbled around in a vain attempt to frame a cogent response; the rest of the class stared hard at the board, as though we might find the answer embedded in the question. Finally a quiet girl named Ann raised her hand.

"Yes, Ann?"

"We look at them? At their faces?"

The professor's face lit up. "That's right," he said. "We observe. We look at their faces."

Simple.

Now, all these years later, I felt the weight of that early lesson. You look, you try to listen, and, through something called the Law of the Interchangeability of Pronouns, you intuit the other's experiences. (The "I-thou relationship" is how existentialist philosopher Martin Buber described the intuitive process. "Me to we" is current usage.) But no one, not even someone as sympathetic as Kitwood, can actually feel another person's pain. Until someone comes up with a new drug or machine or refigured Ouija board that enables advanced dementia patients to communicate their inner life to caregivers, we are all in the dark.

Early stage Lewy Body patients, however, can help by providing a few clues. On the LBDA's online patients' forum, a former psychiatric social worker tried something innovative: he interviewed himself. Playing the double role of patient and psychologist, "dspencer" (his web name) wrote up the results of his clinical self-analysis and offered them up to fellow sufferers:

> Here we are presenting a 63-year-old mwm [married white male] who is in no apparent subjective distress. However, [he] is only oriented to self and not with exactitude to person, time or place.... Affect and verbal process appear much intact, but others complain of mood swings, temper flare-ups, and gross variations in mental and physical activity...

Like The Knitting Doc, dspencer knew his way around the vocabulary. In a second email, he revealed the depth of his loss:

> If I allow myself to forget that I'm so very ill (easy to do, right?), then I discover the many negative behaviors that I hoist onto significant others: neurotic wounding, loss of empathy, anger, paranoid ideation, and an ambiguous sense of loss leading to tearful, painful depression.... The rare beauty of ultra-sensitive insight and ability to heal others is gone like a thief in the night.... I can only see occasional shadows out of the corner of my clinical eye.

I found this patient's description of watching his professional skills going "like a thief in the night" profoundly moving.

CHAPTER 18

Ken, now settled into his sixth-floor hospital room, was no longer "oriented with exactitude to person, time, or place." He hadn't yet reacted to any aspect of the last forty-eight hours. Was he in pain? Did he notice the restraints on his wrists, or the men in the other three beds? Did he know who I was? Who he was?

On the second day of hospitalization, a doctor looked in the door and, seeing me, came in to introduce himself. He asked Ken if he would mind answering a few questions and Ken nodded his willingness.

"Good," the doctor said, smiling encouragingly. "Now, can you tell me what city we are in, Ken?"

"Glasgow."

He wrote a quick note. "Fine. What month it is now?"

"November, I think."

A few more queries and he left. Ken turned to me, something clearly on his mind. "Corry's dead, I guess," he said.

Wow—that startled me. I hastened to reassure him, saying, "No, no, she's fine. Corry's alive and well, very well. I could phone her if you'd like."

"Well do it! Don't just talk about it!"

A fit-looking young woman was the next visitor. "Good morning, Mr. Sobol. I'm Jasmine, your physiotherapist," she said. "We're going to see if we can get you sitting up!"

Ken had been lying prone all morning. When I said that couldn't be good for his internal organs, Jasmine explained that it was more than that: "Your husband has to be able to get himself up and then stay sitting up before we can even think of trying a wheelchair." She worked with him for half an hour, showing him how he could use his stomach muscles to better advantage.

"You can do it, Ken," she urged. "You have the strength. Try again."

Eventually, she got him sitting, propped up with pillows, but it happened mostly through her own considerable muscle power.

"That's okay, Ken," she told him, smiling. "Maybe tomorrow."

She was on her way out the door when he spoke. "Wait!" he called out in a croaky voice.

She turned back, and, standing by his bed, gave him time to gather his thoughts.

"Something very strange happened to me..." he began. "When I was at home...at home...in bed." He stopped, swallowed. "I found I couldn't walk...but then I felt I was being attacked! And I got up...and...and..." He stopped again, unsure how to go on. "And...and I started...I..."

He looked at me for help. I was hesitant about whether he really wanted to hear what happened next. However, when he continued to look at me expectantly, I prompted: "And you got into a bit of a wrestling match with Lori, the care worker. Remember her? That was a first, right? You'd never done anything like that before."

"Yes," he said. "Yes, that's right."

This was the first time Ken had shown any awareness of the early-morning crisis. Did it mean that he trusted Jasmine? I hoped so, because getting him up and active was crucial; and, like anyone, he always responded better to people he liked, people who believed in him.

But no, it turned out I had misread the signs. As soon as Jasmine was out the door, he gestured for me to come close.

"They're out to get us, every single one," he whispered.

"Don't you think some of them might be okay?" I said. "This woman seems very kind. Maybe we can trust her, at least?"

He shook his head, then grabbed my hands and, staring up at me, pressed them together so hard it hurt.

"Every single one!" he cried.

Later, as I sat reading a magazine, he asked of no one in particular, "Is there anyone here who speaks Yiddish or German?" Speaking to an invisible listener or listeners, he explained, "She needs someone who speaks Polish. There must be someone around."

I don't think he means me and there's no other "she" in the room.

One day last winter Ken had become agitated while listening to an online reading of an anti-war play by Caryl Churchill, a writer he usually admires. (A local production of "Top Girls" was one of the last outings we had enjoyed together, before excursions like going to live theater became too difficult for him.) He began mumbling incoherently about "my people" before turning the computer off and walking out of the room. I couldn't tell what exactly had set him off.

Around the same time, as we sat on the streetcar on our way to a medical appointment, he had touched my arm and told me, "That woman over there keeps whispering things to me. Things like, 'Kill all the white men!'" When I looked around and told him I didn't see anything unusual, he indicated a neatly dressed woman who was standing near us and looking out the window, a briefcase in one hand. "Her. I mean *her*," he insisted.

I studied the woman for a moment. She looked deep in thought, maybe about what she was going to say at a big meeting that afternoon.

"Ken, do you think it's possible that you might have misheard her?" I asked him.

"No! I heard her right."

I let it go, but during my next visit to the psychiatric social worker, I brought up the incident. Did she think it possible, I asked, that the woman had actually said something like that to Ken?

"No. Absolutely not, Julie. That story is classic dementia. Absolutely typical," she told me.

That was reassuring in a way, but also extremely depressing. Ever since I'd known Ken he had refused to be typecast, or to typecast others, by race or ethnicity. In cities like London, New York, and Toronto, he had viewed each encounter with a different culture as an opportunity: new foods to try, new maps to study, new insights into the infinitely variable human condition. As recently as his first visit to the day program, where so many clients and staff members hailed from the Azores, he had become intrigued by the history and culture of those windblown islands, coming home one day to announce proudly that he now could count up to ten in Portuguese— not bad for someone with galloping dementia.

It was painful to watch that open attitude, like so many other aspects of his personality, changing: the more so because our own family had, with the arrival of children-in-law and grandchildren, come to resemble a mini–United Nations (Scottish/Jewish/Mexican/African Canadian/Irish/Boer/Quebecois). Living in today's Toronto was that same value writ large.

Over the next few days, whole platoons of specialists stopped by Ken's room to ask questions. A gerontologist explained that they had tested him and that the tests confirmed a severe level of dementia. "Of course," the doctor told me, "that could change as his physical health improves. We can't really predict anything at this stage about what the future looks like. Any physical illness upsets the balance of electrolytes. In the brain of a dementia patient, that means complete havoc. For now it's watch and wait."

The gerontologist was followed by a palliative care team, a movement team, and a pair of social workers, all of whom were remarkably free of the patronizing "white coat" attitude of the doctors I remembered from my childhood. A member of the movement team explained how they might try tinkering with Ken's meds; they might cut back on the Levocarb, might substitute Aricept for Reminyl, might try him again on Seroquel. In this safe hospital setting, I was comfortable with all these possibilities, and sure enough, the tinkering seemed to help.

Within days, Ken's palsy was reduced and his voice improved. Strangely, though the hallucinations were still there—if anything, they had increased in number and variety since his admission—his anxiety about them was lessened. I was happy to see this one source of psychic pain reduced, for however long it lasted.

One morning, I arrived to find a sort of derrick-on-wheels parked at his bedside. "It's called a Hoyer lift," one of the nurses informed me. I watched as Ken, wearing a hospital gown, white legs dangling, was hoisted high above the bed and swung unceremoniously through the air like a load of construction materials. A picture from those congratulatory cards, the ones with a cute drawing of a stork delivering a baby in a sling, flashed into my mind, but Ken took it all calmly enough and the word "back-saving" certainly applied. In no time at all, he was safely deposited in a wheelchair, a blanket tucked around his bare legs.

An aide pushed him down the hall and parked him against the wall directly in front of the nurses' station. I pulled up a chair and here we sat side-by-side once again, except that instead of observing the passing parade from our front porch, we were treated to the kaleidoscopic comings and goings of this floor's busy nerve center. Phones rang continually, nurses conferred, doctors made notes, worried-looking relatives approached the counter to plaintively or aggressively—depending on the family's style—demand satisfactory answers to their questions. Around us, cleaners polished and mopped non-stop.

Ken had by now lost all interest in television, and his conversations with his cheery roommates after the TURP procedure seemed very, very far away. But he needed some form of visual stimulation and this location seemed a good one. Sitting unobserved where you can study people's faces and eavesdrop on their conversations is one of the ways writers have of getting their material—not that Ken had need right now of his once-considerable skill of creating sharp, telling dialogue, but he still carried around a notebook. In it he sometimes jotted down a few words, words that might say anything since they were completely illegible.

Now, each time I emerged from the elevator on his floor, I glanced down the hall to see Ken in his regular spot, watching me as I walked toward him. I never knew what new symptom, or what temporary, illusory improvement I was going to encounter.

"Does he recognize you?" people wanted to know. I told them I wasn't sure. Once in a while, he greeted me with a cheery, "Oh, there you are; I'm glad you've come." But does he really understand that I'm *me*? Or was I just that vaguely familiar woman who visited regularly? I don't think he or anyone else could answer.

Not long after his arrival, one doctor had asked, in front of me, "Who is that lady sitting by your bed, Ken? Can you tell me her name?"

Silence.

After that doctor had left, I had asked him directly.

"Ken, do you know who I am?"

His patience was being tried.

"I don't care *who* you are!"

Our grandchildren, from whom he had always derived so much joy, appeared to be fading from his consciousness. That seemed such a loss, for him and for them. One evening, Corry and Greg's boys, Elliot and Julian, visited. Ken seemed to grasp that these tall young men were his grandsons, but he didn't know their names and had already married off sixteen-year-old Elliot in his mind. (Perhaps it's a matter of how early in life a given memory is implanted; my cousin Carolyn, who has Alzheimer's, greets her two older children by name when they visit, but sadly for the rest of the family, she doesn't recognize the three younger ones.)

One morning, Ken asked as soon as I was within hearing distance, "Is it night yet?" I held up my cellphone to show him the time—11:15 a.m., June 4—and gently reminded him that the date had special significance. He didn't react at first, but when a nurse walked in moments later, he stopped her and said, with a barely discernable touch of pride, "Today's

Jane's birthday. My daughter." Clearly, he retained some sense of our children's identities.

His mood varied day by day as he struggled to make sense of what was happening to him. Mine shifted in reflection of his—either acceptance or tears, depending on how that day's visit went. One afternoon, as we sat together watching the day's developments unfold behind the busy nurses' station, he took a deep breath and turned to me. I had to bend down close to catch the words when he pointed to his chest and whispered in a weak voice, "I can't forget you, Babe, because I keep you in here."

Even then I couldn't be positive I heard him right, but I chose to believe I did. Other family members had their own stories of occasions when Ken's mind emerged from the inner chaos for a few moments of relative lucidity. (I think we all will remember those moments in years to come.)

Hospital visitors look for a way of connecting. The obvious one is finding small ways to be of service, but that's not as easy as it sounds. Ken didn't want to take the elevator down to the busy atrium on the main floor and brushed off my offers to read to him in the same way he had brushed off family members' earlier attempts to enroll him in Dancing with Parkinson's, Aquafit, and an exercise class tailored to people with disabilities. (The Parkinson's choir had been a happy exception to this pattern; he looked forward to practices and did his best at performances.)

If I happened to be there at lunchtime, he did allow me to feed him. He watched intently as I lifted the cover off the plate to reveal what resembled a slab of Neapolitan ice cream, except the three stripes were not strawberry pink, vanilla white, and chocolate brown. One day it might be an unappealing palette of orange, pale green, and tan (puréed squash, peas, and chicken); on other days, stripes of beige, dark green, and white (puréed beef, spinach, mashed potato). So far, he hadn't commented on the fact he was eating a soft diet; he never took his eyes off me as I dipped into one of the stripes and moved a pale green spoonful toward his mouth. Once it was swallowed, I filled the spoon again, brought it back empty. The action, repeated over and over, felt almost intimate.

One morning, Ken indicated that he wanted to try feeding himself. When the number of spoonfuls that reached his mouth outnumbered the bright splotches on the bib covering his chest, it felt like another of those small but not-so-small victories.

A few days later, a young woman I'd never seen before approached me in the hall where I sat waiting for the nurses to finish with Ken's morning routine. "Do you have a moment?" she asked. She introduced herself as Susan, the hospital's CCAC liaison person, and she was eager to tell me about a program the provincial government was putting together, one that she said might make it possible for Ken to return home.

I was caught off guard. We had been warned early on that we should do everything possible to avoid this situation; I had heard stories from people about their relatives ending up in long-term facilities outside the city, languishing there for months before something closer to home was found for them. We were lucky that this hospital was a short streetcar ride from our home, though a busy surgical ward wasn't the right place for Ken; at best, patients like him fall between every set of tracks in the rail yard. I'd looked into hospice care and been told that it was not an option—though anyone could see that Ken was very ill, there was always the possibility he could hang on for years, and hospice beds are intended for patients who are closer to the end.

So I listened to Susan's glowing description of the "Ageing at Home" plan, but it sounded too much like a vacuum cleaner sales pitch to be convincing. Every time I attempted to describe our failed attempt at home care—the attack on Lori, and the catheter disaster—it brought on another paean to the program's advantages. Partial payment for hospital bed rental! More hours of personal care! These sounded fine as far as they went, but the offer was somehow detached from our family's reality, as though Ken's multi-faceted needs, and my health, were annoying irrelevancies. Susan got up to leave. Smiling, she handed me some literature. "Just think it over, Julie," she insisted. "I'll be in touch soon to talk again."

I phoned Zoe, the social worker associated with Ken's geriatrician, as she had proved helpful before. She listened to my story, then told me, "You do not have to accept this offer. People can turn it down. You have that choice." That was good to know, but I needed time to mull this over. Ken was a person, not a misdirected mail order.

I tried the hospital social worker. Sheila had worked in the field for decades and was familiar with all the ins and outs. At our first meeting, she had questioned me in detail about Ken's symptoms, her eyes widening when she heard my description of the wrestling scene. That day she had advised categorically, "Listen to me. Do *not* let them try to talk you into taking him home again." Today, when I reached her, she repeated that same advice.

Quick calls to each of our kids. In the end, our family, with some regret, formed a united front with the two social workers: I rejected the Ageing at Home offer. A few hours later Sheila phoned me to say the hospital had discussed the case, and they would be allowing Ken to stay.

We were all relieved. The CCAC can only do so much with its limited funding, and Ken's care in hospital had been good, or as good as the busy nurses could manage. If there was blame to be placed for situations like this—of which there will be more and more as the population ages—it's on our society as a whole. Science has artificially extended the human life span, but society hasn't yet faced head-on the consequences of that change. We don't place enough value on caregiving in all its forms, professional and informal, and we refuse to question our Western obsession with extending life at any cost.

CHAPTER 19

"All the doctors say I'm getting better! Each one of them has okayed my going home! So you can take me now!"

My tug-of-war with the CCAC rep wasn't witnessed by Ken, but perhaps he heard the staff discussing his case. Now he wanted to go home. His feelings were not hard to understand, but he was still bleeding from having ripped out the catheter, and even here in the hospital, surrounded by caregivers, there had been a couple of falls. One day, he had astonished the nurses by maneuvering himself out of bed and staggering as far as the door before collapsing. "I was hiking up north," he had told me later. "Even though I was from the south, and it was way too cold for me. I may have fainted."

"I know you'd like to be at home," I told him each time he repeated his request. "I wish it could be managed. But look what happened when you came home before. And right now you need good medical care." That reasoning worked for a little while.

One day, though, as we sat together, he suddenly became agitated. "I don't know what we have in common any more!" He was very angry. "I'm so mad I'll…I don't know what I'll do…"

I couldn't listen any more. I stood up to leave.

"I'll…I'll divorce you!" he called after me as I fled to the elevator, ignoring the stares of other patients and visitors.

Back at home, I sifted through our CDs. Rosanne Cash's "Sea of Heartbreak" duet with Bruce Springsteen wasn't a bad match for my bleak mood; nothing like an all-out blues number to make you feel better. When the album finished, I was ready for a good walk. I circled the block, eventually wandering into the corner park. The afternoon sun was beating down, and there wasn't much shade, so I found an empty bench near the wading pool. The park was crowded with mothers and toddlers. Watching the small jostling kids splash each other and pretend to swim ("Watch me, Mom! I'm swimming! Look! Mom? You're not *looking*!"), I felt vicariously cooled. From time to time, drops of the churning water landed on my pathetically grateful feet.

My thoughts were far away as out of the corner of my eye I saw two young women approaching the bench. I slid over to make room, but when one of them bumped up against me and the other laughed, I glanced up.

It was my daughters, all smiles and a sight for sore eyes.

It was a day in mid-June, when Ken, after studying the activity at the nurses' desk, volunteered, "Some of these people are champion fighters, you know. They can get pretty violent sometimes."

I put down my paper. It was a typical day on the ward, everyone busy with the usual phone calls, conferences, and form filling. Every so often, a nurse would jump up from her paperwork and run to help when a second or third pair of hands was needed somewhere. A better example of teamwork would be hard to imagine.

No wonder the nurses had begun to work their way into Ken's hallucinations. They seemed to be everywhere at once, such a big part of any hospital scene and a major focus in fictional portraits of hospital life, TV shows like *Scrubs* and *E.R.* What was strange, however, was his tone. As casually as if he were telling me that he had been served ice cream for lunch, he informed me that one of the nurses had killed a co-worker that morning.

"And there's a man who's always hiding in the bathroom," he added. "Now what's his name…Price, I think—something like that. A classic hit man."

"You mean, he was waiting in the shower room? This hit man?"

Laughing, he gently corrected me. "No, no. Not in the shower. In the *bathroom*. What would he be doing in the *shower?*"

Of course. The bathroom, not the shower. Despite the gravity of the situation, I had to laugh with him.

On a different morning, he commented, "There are three sisters that look alike. I can't tell the difference between the three, though I know you're one of them."

"Really?" I replied, feeling cautiously pleased.

He nodded. "Yes. And one of the sisters is nicer than the others."

"I hope I'm the nice one."

"Not exactly. But you are nice."

A few years back the papers ran a story about a popular Canadian comic who kept insisting, to anyone who would listen, that his young wife and baby had been spirited away and replaced by decoys; she was so alarmed by his rants that she took the baby and ran. A psychiatrist called into court identified the problem as Capgras, a little-known condition that affects the mind's ability to connect memory and emotion, causing the afflicted person to believe their loved one, friend, or parent has been replaced by an identical-looking imposter.

That was the first time I had heard of the condition. Since then, I had come across occasional references in my reading about LBD and heard of a couple of instances closer to home. The father of our artist friend, Gary, was convinced Gary's mother had just returned to the family home after running away with another man and staying away for years. (In reality, she had never left.) The father of another acquaintance complained that he never knew which of his two wives—the good one and the bad one—he was going to find when he walked into a room.

Until the three sisters story, though, I had somehow never connected Ken with the syndrome. The floaters he spoke of after the TURP, the "other house" delusions, the duplicates of me he described seeing during his week in short-term care, now made better sense to me, once I saw them for what they were: Capgras doublings. If I had understood that earlier, I might have been better equipped to handle that last frantic search, by the dim light of the streetlamps, for the house that wasn't there.

But hindsight is never very helpful; what *was* helping these days was that for the first time in years, I was getting some solid sleep. The first few nights after Ken went to the hospital I had continued to awaken around four a.m., and often stayed awake. Then one morning, the clock insisted I'd been out cold for eleven hours. Since then, it was like coming across an oasis after wandering for days in the desert with an empty canteen; I couldn't drink deeply enough.

As I began to feel more rested, pieces of life's daily puzzle fell into place more easily. I noticed how much the disease had infiltrated every aspect of our daily life. How restorative, now, was the fact that ordinary household objects—chairs, tables, carpets, coat racks, doors, windows, shower nozzles—had returned to just being themselves and were no longer seen as a threat, as Ken had insisted. Sleep is wonderful stuff.

And in the hospital, the life lessons continued for me. As one day led to the next, my feelings for Ken, as we sat side-by-side in our usual spot, were changing. This new cluster of emotions included a different kind of tenderness, one completely lacking in judgment. Sometimes it felt as if we were not so much husband and wife as comrades in a war not of our choosing.

With more time on my hands, I also began to wonder, given recent findings about the brain's neuroplasticity, if it was possible that Ken was more cognizant of things than I thought. Could it be that he, like our friend Gwen, had consolations of which I was not aware—occasional memory flashes of happier days, some slight sense of private battles won in his daily struggle, of small kindnesses shown by nurses and other workers during the long hospital days and nights? I hoped so.

Among our boxes of family photos, there was one of Ken at age two or so, being held in the arms of his beaming mother. That happy family scene wouldn't last, but it was real at that moment and I felt a momentary compassion for those young parents (now long dead). What emotional struggle would they go through if they could see their son in his present vulnerable state?

I was also becoming more aware of the subtle but very present compensations that caregiving affords. (Nurses and personal care workers sometimes speak of this phenomenon, but it applies to non-professionals, too.) In this all-out age of the individual, the simple act of forcing yourself to slow down, working to find the emotional rhythm of the other person, can be beneficial. Tom Kitwood goes further. He believes that dementia patients, because they lack the inhibitions of polite society, are asking us all "to heal the rift in experience that Western culture has engendered and inviting us to return to aspects of our being that are much older in evolutionary terms: more in tune with the body and its functions, closer to the life of instinct."

Despite the fact that Ken seldom spoke these days, and that when he did it was brief and often accompanied by anger, I sometimes got the feeling that he was trying to teach me something. I wanted to be a good pupil, so what specific lesson was he teaching? Perhaps something along the lines of:

Words don't tumble out as they used to, so please don't expect too much of me.

Try to make sense of my ramblings: I still crave human company.

Look me in the eye, but please don't touch me: I need privacy.

If my rules confuse you, ignore them. Just sit with me for a while.

Be still. Consider before you speak. Shhh.

June 21: This morning I overheard some of the hospital staff talking about the upcoming G20 meetings in Toronto. Apparently a rumor was going round that patients might be moved out in preparation for trouble on the street. The prediction struck me as one of those over-the-top stories that circulate before any big event, but I was concerned about the possibility of the effect on Ken if it were true.

In the afternoon, I attended Ximena's kindergarten graduation with William. As we enjoyed some post-ceremony cake and lemonade in the schoolyard, two outsized khaki-painted helicopters passed overhead. The kids looked up briefly and returned to their games, but the roar drowned out all adult conversation. As the low-flying copters moved out of sight, one mother looked up and commented scornfully: "Do they think we're hiding bombs in their diapers?" Just at that moment Ximena, spotting us from across the yard, gave me a wave and her friend Pedro smiled shyly in my direction.

Boarding a streetcar, two days later, I spotted a free seat and eased into it with relief. We had only traveled a few blocks when the driver braked sharply. "Sorry, folks, I can't take you any farther. The street's blocked." Joining the other passengers on the sidewalk, I could hear boisterous cheering off to my left. Turning to look, I saw a large demonstration snaking its way down the busy street. There were more cheers as a young man with a bullhorn yelled encouragement.

I had seen protests like this in other cities, and had participated in a few of them, but this was larger than any I had witnessed personally, in New York or Montreal or anywhere else. I couldn't see to the end of the crowd. And something else struck me as odd: on this early summer day in the orderly city of Toronto, for every man, woman and child shuffling peacefully past the coffee shops and computer stores that line the street, there was at least one policeman standing in a parallel line by the curb.

The mood was friendly enough, for now. The two rows of this urban line dance—protesters looking a bit wilted in the heat but still upbeat and energized, cops in their dark blue twill attempting to appear stern and tolerant at the same time—mostly just ignored each other. And you expect a police presence at any mass event, that's a given. But it was a question of proportion, and this scene came much too close to giving the appearance of martial law.

Talk about the summit built over the next few days. Theater openings were being cancelled, dinner parties put on hold. A three-game series between the Blue Jays and the Phillies was moved to safety in Philadelphia. Wherever I went, there was someone with an opinion they want me to hear. Meanwhile, hospital staff and social workers were scanning the city in search of alternative bed space for, among others, Ken Sobol.

In the car after an afternoon jazz recital, Corry and I stared at the sea of placards bobbing above the heads of a large crowd around the provincial legislative buildings. The signs were too far away to make out so I turned on the car radio and listened in disbelief as the announcer spoke of smashed windows and fistfights. Back home I turned on the TV and watched demonstrators being beaten by helmeted, booted Arms-ageddon cops, police cars on fire, chaos on the streets of Toronto. It felt to me as if the city itself were splintering in pieces.

By the next morning there was much talk of "anarchists" and something called the Black Bloc. "What's your reaction to the trouble-makers?" reporters kept asking people. I boarded a bus to see with my own eyes what was happening.

When I got off at the stop across the street from the legislative buildings, I walked past a local poverty activist who was being interviewed by an alternative TV station. Otherwise, this part of the park was quiet except for a few people wandering around looking slightly lost. Over in one corner of the grounds a group of policemen stood in a circle conferring seriously. One of them glanced over at me briefly, then turned back; I didn't look suspicious enough for questioning. A cluster of young people who could have been tourists or protestors or undercover cops, for all I knew, huddled together near some flowerbeds. Evidently the main action had moved closer to the city center.

Though it was still early, the day was already turning into a scorcher. I found an empty bench under one of the big trees. Somewhere above me a bird tweeted his song. The leaves of the maples stirred in the light breeze. *Peace.* I closed my eyes for a minute. It felt good to be away for a short while from the narrow world of back and forthing between home and hospital.

This brief respite was so restorative, that I opted for a bit more exploring before heading home.

Near the legislature's front doors, I chatted with an older man who had a couple of fancy-looking cameras looped around his neck. He told me he had already been stopped several times and asked for identification, though with his neat appearance and all that expensive gadgetry, he didn't look like any kind of anarchist. I moved on. In another far corner marked as a "designated speech area," I spotted what looked like some action. Maybe the activists had decided there should continue to be a limited presence in the area.

Up close, though, this was a clot of black-clad, bearded rabbis who were holding a completely peaceful protest of their own. No burning of cop cars here; instead, lots of praying. After I stood observing for a while, I decided it wouldn't be rude to approach one of them and explain my curiosity about their connection to the G20 meeting.

The man was happy to talk. "We're not here because of the G20," he explained, as his fellow protesters continued to daven back and forth in prayer. "No, we're not concerned with what's happening in Toronto. We are here today to publicly express our conviction that politics has no place in the realm of religion. The two should be kept completely separate."

I told him I agreed with him (though likely for slightly different reasons). Thanking him for his time and his courtesy, I turned and headed home, leaving the quiet green space to the squirrels, the tourists, the stern-looking cops, the alternative tv crews, and the prayerful rabbis.

By evening a new expression, "kettling," had entered the city's vocabulary. The word, with its hint of confinement, of emotions building inside a hot, uncomfortable space, has a sinister sound. During a torrential downpour, a solid phalanx of police had surrounded a crowd of perhaps two hundred—many of them, it would later turn out, ordinary citizens on their way to a meeting or a party. If there were one or two anarchists among the tightly packed crowd as the heavy rain pelted their heads, slid down their faces, and soaked into their clothes, they had to be as miserable as everyone else on my wide-screen TV.

After much huffing and showing of press cards, a few journalists caught in the crowd were allowed to leave unharmed (if dampish), but their presence made for fascinating television. Perhaps it wasn't a coincidence that coverage of the next day's events was more thoughtful and in-depth.

The final tally? Three police cars set on fire, dozens of stores vandalized, and more than a thousand people held for questioning, of whom 714 were taken into custody. There was also one happy statistic. Deaths: 0. Buildings destroyed: 0.

CHAPTER 20

The next morning I found the hospital doors locked, but I was allowed to enter after assuring the guard I was there to visit my sick husband. With the visiting heads of state returning to their respective countries and the demonstrators and visiting policemen back at their regular jobs, the city was settling down.

Up on the sixth floor it was always pleasantly cool, no matter how hot it got down on the street. When I impulsively took off my broad-brimmed sun hat and put it on Ken's head as a joke, a couple of the nurses glanced across the counter and smiled. A young orderly called out, "Lookin' good, Ken," as he walked by. Ken looked pleased at these reactions—a good sign, indicating his vanity had not completely deserted him.

But he wasn't lookin' good. John, on his last visit, had

taken a few shots with his digital camera. Ken's face in the photos, when John handed the camera to me for a look, was so gaunt and gray and stern that for a couple of seconds my mind didn't register the evidence of my eyes. The weight loss had altered the familiar angles of his face, and on his hands he was wearing what looked like huge white boxing gloves, a replacement for the restraints that he had managed to pull off a few times.

On second look, I found that having these images to hold and study brought Ken closer to me. In this visual, digital, technological age, taking pictures is what we do, and this was what his face looked like now. The weight loss, though, was worrisome. His weight had been going down over the winter and had continued to drop in the hospital. On Father's Day, when Corry brought him a smoked meat sandwich, he had finished it down to the last crumb of rye, the last salty shred of tasty beef. But the other day, he had a coughing fit while I was feeding him. When I offered him water, a nurse had quickly looked over at us and shook her head. A swallowing test was ordered and the results were bothersome enough that a second test was arranged for the next day. For this one, they would use a special x-ray video camera.

I could hear the concern in the speech therapist's voice when she phoned me at home after the second test. The results had been conclusive, she said. The staff would be changing his feeding regime; she would leave explanatory brochures at the desk for me. This new development was discouraging and hard to absorb. John, over the phone that evening, said I sounded tired.

A few days ago, the CCAC told me I could add two names to our list of preferred residences. I visited a few places and found two in the downtown area that seemed possible. I added them to the list, and waited.

Ken had still not complained about the change in his diet, but he had become pale and uncommunicative. I needed someone to give me a picture of the overall state of his health; with different medical teams in constant movement around the various hospital floors, I had lost track of which name went with which face and which face with which specialty. Even if I were one of those efficient people who writes everything down in a little book, there was still the challenge of tracking each specialist down or reaching them by phone. This morning one helpful doctor asked me, "Has no one told you about our 'family meetings' yet?" At any point in time, he explained, just by speaking to a nurse, I could have summoned forth whichever staff members I wanted to speak with and a meeting would have been arranged. I quickly put the wheels in motion for a family meeting, specifying the presence of his speech therapist and physiotherapist.

On July 9, Corry, and I met with Carolyn (the speech pathologist), Ryan (one of Ken's physiotherapists), and the resident on duty.

"See that? See that small smudge right there?" Carolyn asked, pointing to her laptop. We were seated around the table in a small, nondescript room near the nurses' desk. I obediently craned my neck for a closer look.

"Watch," she began again, pointing at an x-ray video of someone's jaw chewing food. "See the dark spot moving down? Right there? That's food going down the wrong passageway. It's happening a lot. Not huge amounts, but still not good." This graphic image made its point when words had not. At first I assumed this was a general-purpose educational film, until Corry leaned over and whispered, "Mom, those are Dad's glasses!"

Carolyn then moved quickly into a brief lesson on the anatomy of the human throat, pointing out the larynx, pharynx, and trachea before emphasizing again the danger of even small particles of food causing an infection as they accumulated in the lungs. That aside, of course, a more immediate danger was choking.

Food had been the last real intimacy. I had enjoyed bringing Ken small treats, breaking off tiny bits of a chocolate bar or feeding him, very slowly, one juicy blueberry at a time. He was so eager for whatever was on offer that his pleasure in these occasional indulgences made me enjoy them, too. That's finished now: no more chocolate, no blueberries—and certainly no more smoked meat sandwiches.

Ken wouldn't even be allowed to enjoy a drink of cold water when he was thirsty. All liquids, Carolyn explained, would from now on be mixed with a product called ThickenUp to lessen the likelihood of drops sliding into his airway. She noticed my dismayed reaction and told me, "It could be worse. Of the three types of thickening this company provides—nectar, honey, and pudding—Mr. Sobol has only reached the honey level. If and when his condition worsens we'll have to move him to the pudding level." Drinking something that has the consistency of pudding sounded like a form of torture, not on level with waterboarding (a personal nightmare) but bad enough.

"What about walking?" I asked. "Will he ever walk again? Really walk, I mean, not just the few steps he's taken along the hallway." Ryan, the physiotherapist, shook his head. "You shouldn't get your hopes up. It's not a question of strength— Mr. Sobol is strong enough. But walking is a very complex action. Right now, it's hard for his brain to put together all the different variables."

We had already told the hospital that we wouldn't opt for tubal feeding. Corry asked the team to expand a bit on the implications of that decision. "According to recent studies," Carolyn replied, "feeding tubes don't extend the life of dementia patients. In fact, since the tubes are a potential source of infection, they may actually shorten the person's life."

Her answer helped confirm our earlier choice.

Med schools must be interesting places to be around these days, I thought. Social change happens slowly, as a rule, but it's obvious that certain difficult ethical issues are being addressed more openly than in the past. I left this meeting feeling profoundly grateful for the candor of these medical professionals, all young enough to be my children. They had clearly thought things over before they sat down with us, and had answered our questions frankly.

With Ken no longer able to articulate his needs, access to straight talk (from both a medical and human viewpoint) was essential. But, I wondered, do doctors ever get used to patients and their families asking all the hard questions?

(Years back, Ken and I had discussed some of these end-of-life issues; at one point, he had even written up his own version of a living will. It read as follows: "If a hospital decides any of my organs can be successfully transplanted into someone else, that's fine with me. However, I do find that eventuality pretty hard to imagine. After all, if they were that good I'd still be alive.")

Someone had shaved off the small beard Ken was growing, leaving him with a dapper-looking Charlie Chaplin mustache. Jane told me that yesterday when she visited he wanted to know where I was. "Is she out of the country?" he wanted to know. "Here I am," I pointed out when I arrived this morning.

When I suggested a long walk—in his case, a ride—he didn't seem sure about it. But he didn't object as we set off through the white-painted, mostly empty corridors. I pushed the chair up the ramp leading into another wing, and down a series of hallways that brought us out into the ophthalmology wing. The TV in the waiting room was turned on to a World Cup match. I suggested watching for a while, thinking he might enjoy the world championship of a sport he had played in college.

"No," he responded. "I want to go back. Let's go."

Back we rolled through the maze of hallways. A wrong turn at one corner meant negotiating a U-turn in a narrow space.

"They're going to put me in jail," he said gloomily once I had us on our way again. "I'll need you to be my backup."

"Yes, fine," I said. "I can do that. But I thought I already was. Your backup, I mean."

"No, you haven't been."

I tried diversion.

"Ken, do you remember my saying that Rick Arnold is coming to see you tomorrow? He's driving all the way in from Bolton."

"Yes. But Rick's in on it, too."

We had reached the nurses' desk.

"I haven't killed anyone, have I?" he asked.

"No, you haven't killed anyone. And you haven't robbed anyone either. You're a good person. You haven't done any of those things."

Before I left, I reminded him I'd be back in the morning. He shook his head. "No, they won't let you in," he said. "We'll never see each other anymore."

He is so far gone now, I thought to myself as I walked home. In a sense, there was (almost) no one there. Yet some part of him remained. And outside the hospital, life trundled on, as it had to.

The next day, Ken was asleep when I arrived around eleven. This was unusual; typically, between the hustle and bustle of the morning ablutions, and the hospital's strict routine, patients have trouble sleeping in late. The young nurse at his bedside looked up as I entered and told me they had been trying to wake him up with no success. "We've sent for the doctor," she added.

He was still asleep when Rick showed up at eleven thirty. We stood together by his bedside, looking down at him. Though his wide shoulders still had some muscle, his body looked so shrunken under the thin blanket. When Rick tried saying hello, Ken's eyes fluttered open briefly and then closed.

I managed to get a few words out; his eyes half opened again. Now he wanted to say something.

I leaned in close to hear.

"Please stop talking," he said.

The nurse had trouble inserting the IV needle. An older woman got it done easily when she was called in. With all the poking and prodding, Ken was starting to appear more alert. The two women helped him sit up, and suddenly he was wide awake and ready to talk. Rick launched into a reminiscing session about their student days in London, encouraging Ken when he lost the thread of the conversation. *Moore, Duckworth, Tsum Pei.* Familiar names. I left them to it.

Later, over lunch, Rick told me, "You know, I really enjoyed seeing Ken. I keep a list of people for whom I pray every morning, and you two are among the names on it. I ask for help for 'JulieKen'—that's how I think of the two of you."

Rick was well aware that Ken and I both kept our distance from organized religion, but I was touched. No one in recent years had asked for divine intervention on my behalf, or if they had, they hadn't made a point of telling me. But if I'm going to be prayed for, Rick is the person to do it. A man of his word.

When I walked through the door after returning home from lunch, the phone was ringing. Was I still interested in placing Ken in Kensington? a woman at the CCAC wanted to know. Because a room had just become available. He could move in tomorrow.

"Yes," I answered. "Yes, we are still interested."

The hospital staff had done their best, but nurses on the surgery ward are not trained in dementia caregiving, and the right person for the right illness is a pretty basic rule of medicine.

The sun is shining, oh happy day. I picked up the phone again to let Corry know.

CHAPTER 21

Subject: Really good news!
Date: July 13, 2010
To: jane sobol, william sanchez, louis sobol, john sobol, annie hillis, greg clarke, julian, elliot

Hi, everyone,
Great news: Dad/Grandpa will be moving into Kensington Gardens tomorrow afternoon!

I just got off the phone with Mom, and she's so, so glad that it's worked out like this—our best-case scenario for Dad's care.

(You may want to hold off for a little bit [before phoning]. She said she was going to lie down—the day started off rather hairy, though everything is fine now.)

Dad will have his own room where he can have quiet, privacy and his own furnishings/homey things, and it'll be so much better for visits, too. In the end, he'll have a shared washroom, which is actually a good thing because it reduces the monthly costs quite a bit, but he still gets a private room.

Kensington is about a four-minute walk from our place, and most importantly, it's so close for Mom, and for Jane, too!

I just had dinner this week with a friend whose mother has been in the dementia ward at Kensington for several years, and they have been really happy with the level of care and the staff.

Tomorrow I'll go to the hospital at 1 p.m. to get things ready, and then Dad and I will ride by ambulance to Kensington and get him settled in.

Talk to you soon,
Corry

Corry's email had said it all. And now here was Ken, comfortably ensconced in his own pleasant second-floor room, the windows of which faced onto a small courtyard. I felt very fortunate; this facility had been one of our original choices and was within walking distance of the house. When he first arrived this morning he was disoriented, not surprising given that he had been dislodged from now-familiar surroundings and loaded once more into an ambulance for another ride across town. He looked more comfortable after a nap, even seeming to have some awareness of his surroundings.

That evening, John and Annie came by the house, having driven down from Ottawa. They had stopped in first to see Ken. John reported that they were greeted enthusiastically and that Ken informed them, pointing to a photograph we'd placed on his dresser, "That's Julian with his girlfriend!"

"Before we left," Annie added, "he took our hands in his and spoke affectionately—almost like a kind of blessing. He was great!"

And on the following morning, I found Ken dressed! Feeding himself! Cooperative! Seated at a table in the dining room! I couldn't believe it. His three lunch companions were a man whose Pan-Africa t-shirt in Rasta colors bore the nametag "Goodwill" and two women, Gertrude and Eleanora. Judging from their careful posture and quiet manner, I guessed the pair might be retired schoolteachers. A worker brought a chair and I sat down to enjoy the welcome sight of Ken in this normalized setting. I couldn't believe it.

Goodwill had given me a friendly nod as I joined the party, but otherwise no one spoke much; they were all intent on their food.

"Mrs. Sobol?"

I glanced up. A tall, rather serious-looking man was staring down at me. "I'm Randy, Ken's dietician. Thought I'd stop by and introduce myself."

We shook hands. I remarked on how everyone was really digging in—literally—to their lunches. "Yes," he said. "I used to work in a hospital, and there's no comparison. Here you get real food. We really make an effort."

He glanced over at Ken, who had finished his meal and

was now reaching across the table for Gertrude's juice. Randy quickly moved the glass out of reach.

"I wanted to speak to you about liquids," he went on. "A bit of water's not necessarily a problem. I mean, of course people can drown from too much water, but we all swallow saliva—we do it all the time. Really, the main thing is that he eat slowly."

He glanced again at Ken, frowning. "He's supposed to have just a teaspoon to eat with—to slow him down. I'll speak to someone."

It was sobering to be reminded of the swallowing issue so soon, but they seemed more relaxed about it here than at the hospital. Ken had managed to feed himself, and as I pushed him back to his room, he actually waved at a couple of other residents. Perhaps, I thought, just perhaps, his health would improve enough in this new, welcoming setting that we might manage an occasional outing. We might even try a home visit. The postcard hope was still there.

The building got lots of light from many of its windows, and there was greenery behind every one of them. Its layout was simple: bedrooms on three sides of a U-shaped corridor; staff offices in the windowless middle area. On the fourth side, one door led to the elevator lobby, another to the lunchroom. During our earlier tours of various facilities, I had noticed that many of the residents had computers in their room. Here on the dementia ward, however, I didn't spot a single computer. It seemed decades ago that the family had discussed buying one for the day (which I then thought of as being in the distant future) when Ken moved into a residence.

Most patients did have TVs in their rooms, but few sets were switched on. In the dayroom, though, several wheelchairs were parked in front of a large set. Some residents had nodded off; a few stared silently as a newsreader related the latest stories and a crawl across the screen reaffirmed her words. One resident nodded hello to Ken as we arrived, then quickly moved his eyes back to the TV.

I left him there for awhile and continued my walk around the floor, stopping to study the contents of a small, glassed-in cupboard outside one room. I had seen these "memory boxes" before, in some of the newer facilities. I didn't know whether the patients paid any attention to them, but perhaps some did. If so, just the fact their families had taken the time to pick out a few special things and bring them in must have what they call a "life-affirming" effect. This particular display, like many, included snapshots of grandchildren and a formal wedding photo of a smiling couple in clothes dating from the early Fifties.

I checked out a few more of the personal mini histories. Some families had included an artifact of special significance—a hand-painted scroll with Chinese characters, a piece of intricate embroidery, a stuffed animal, an athletic award, a floral teacup and saucer, a doll. While I was studying a box in which the only thing on display was a small sign that had likely once hung in a shop window ("Shoes Repaired Here"), two staff members stopped by to chat. Miriam, the older of the two, was the nurse on day duty. Marta explained she would be Ken's personal care worker. We spoke a bit about Ken, and about the various activities available. I liked them both.

Tom Kitwood, in his book on dementia care, wasn't all gloom and doom. He wrote about the vast improvements he had seen since the early days, and described what he imagined long-term residences could be in the future. He envisioned a place so reassuring that even residents who weren't quite sure where they were wouldn't be nervous or fearful. Essential to his plan was a flowering garden. New patients strolling its welcoming paths, he wrote, would gradually become aware of other people in the garden:

Several of them seem to know you; it is a joy to be greeted so warmly, and by name. There are one or two of them whom you feel sure you know well...As you pass by a mirror you catch a glimpse of a person who looks quite old. Is it your grandmother or that person who used to live next door? Anyway, it is good to see her, too.... Her hand is held out toward you, waiting for you to grasp it. As you talk together, the fear evaporates like the morning mist, and you are again in the garden, relaxing in the golden warmth of the sun.

Over the last few years, architects and designers have been edging closer to that vision. Kensington had a front courtyard with benches and flowering bushes. In back of the building there was a larger space where residents could grow their own flowers and vegetables. Historic photos of this neighborhood, where many of the building's residents had grown up, hung on the walls. The downstairs parlor featured a large decorative birdcage where tiny, brightly colored birds warbled as they swooped back and forth all day. One of residence's brochures boasted, "The very essence of all that we try to do in the home is to preserve the kind of normal life that the resident is accustomed to enjoying.... Residents thrive when they are given even the smallest challenges, such as making food or clothing choices, or the responsibility of tending a plant or caring for a pet."

I don't doubt the stories of neglect I've read about certain privately run residences. We need a tightening up of regulations, backed by government inspectors who know what to look for. But many nursing homes are neither hellholes nor luxurious palaces. Some seniors say they prefer the security, companionship, and group outings available at a residence over staying home alone. According to a study of four Vancouver facilities ("Moving into a Nursing Home: A guide for Families" by Peter Silin) 75 percent of residents said they don't feel lonely. Eighty percent even reported they often felt happy.

The painful truth is that advanced dementia holds a person prisoner no matter what the setting. The new pills help—if patients are willing to take them—but not that much. What matters more is kindness, good food, attention to basic physical needs, and a range of leisure activities on offer. In the provincially run residences I had visited, I met many caregivers (like Miriam and Marta) who obviously loved their work and tried to make sure their patients got the best possible care. Much also depends on the proximity of relatives to the facility, and on family willingness to continue playing an active role in the patient's life.

Beyond good hiring practices and adequate funding, large institutions of any kind—hospitals, schools, long-term residences—need to find small practical ways to improve their environment. In long-term care facilities, that includes resident-tended gardens, memory boxes that serve as visual reminders, private dining rooms where families can celebrate special occasions, and communal laundry rooms where even young grandchildren can help Grandma or Grandpa with their weekly washing. Simple and not expensive innovations like these offer alternatives to mindless TV watching or one more forced conversation about the weather.

Kensington Gardens, like many of the newer residences, has one of these private dining rooms. If things went well, perhaps we could put it to use next month for our fiftieth anniversary party.

The next morning I gathered up a copy of Ken's Babe Ruth biography, a photo of me that he likes (though I don't), and a glass insulator from our country auction days; I put them in a bag for Annie so she could arrange them for him when she visited that afternoon. Later that day, I met her, and several other family members, in a park downtown. We spread a blanket and settled down to enjoy an al fresco takeout meal.

After a few minutes, Annie put down her crispy tofu. "Ken talked a lot today," she began, "especially when we were doing the memory box." I was all ears, waiting to hear more about how the day went. "He commented on the photo, Julie. And he watched while I was arranging the other stuff. Oh, he waved hello to another client in the hall. That seemed promising. We chatted for a while about this and that, and then all of a sudden it was, 'You can go now.' So I did."

She picked up her plate, then immediately put it down

again. "Oh, I just remembered. He had a comment about your artist friend Gary. He told me, 'Gary's gone all weird these days.'"

Good-natured laughter all around. Everyone knew that if Ken were here as his old self, he would be laughing louder than anybody. I could almost hear him saying, "Look who's talking."

Office workers carrying their suit jackets over their arms cut through the sun and shade of the pathways on the way home from work, kids rode by on bikes and skateboards, and not far from where we were sitting, a softball game was getting underway. It was a beautiful evening.

Marta, who frets about the air conditioning, yesterday requested six old-fashioned sleeveless undershirts for Ken. I drove to a nearby mall and found a store that actually stocked them. When I took the shirts in, I found him sitting up in bed, looking more perky than I had seen him in months. "I'm so glad you're here," he told me.

Here, in a place where everyone either has dementia or is familiar with the disease, it was easier to relate to him one-on-one, as a person rather than a collection of symptoms. And how lovely it was to see his personal characteristics emerge just a bit from wherever they had been hiding.

When Marta stopped by later, he bantered with her and she replied in kind. As she turned to leave, she told him, "Ken, you're having a good morning."

A few days later, I arrived to find him up on his feet, being helped down the hall by an aide who offered the self-evident statement, "We're working on his mobility."

Back in the hospital, I had witnessed one successful experiment with using a walker. His face had lit up when I told him afterward how great it was to see up him and about. That kind of thing was so rare, an open look of pleasure— although maybe it was just the eye of the beholder. I kept remembering a leisurely stroll up Broadway with friends one fall day in 1959, all the way from lower Manhattan up to Times Square. At the age of twenty-two, you feel you could just keep walking on and on, round the world and back again. Since then, Ken and I had walked our way across many other urban neighborhoods and down numerous country roads where, at every other farm or so, a dog would run out, barking ferociously, to the end of the laneway, only to stop and wag its tail when it finally reached you. I didn't like the idea of all that pleasure coming to a complete end.

The early morning attack that had left Ken weak and wheelchair-bound had never been definitely diagnosed, though a small stroke (one which would not necessarily have shown up in an EKG) was considered a strong possibility. Whatever the cause, I understood that it was hard for his brain to coordinate all the systems needed for walking. And I knew that people could live good lives in a wheelchair; just look at Gwen. Still, the overall quality of Ken's life was so hard to watch. It wasn't just that he couldn't walk, or manage the toilet, or take a bath on his own. It was that he also couldn't eat real food or enjoy a cold beer with friends, or go shopping or see a play or take in a ball game. He didn't watch TV and had stopped responding to music, couldn't rock and roll in any sense of the phrase.

However, I was happy to notice, he appeared to be cooperating with the aide's attempt to help him regain a degree of mobility. And now that his cognition had improved a bit here, and if his walking also got better, shouldn't that have a cumulative good effect on his overall health? During a long illness, any improvement should matter.

After twenty minutes on his feet, Ken needed to rest. Back in his room, Marta looked in to check on the laundry. As she tidied the shelves, she mentioned that yesterday she had left him sitting alone in the wheelchair, and when she returned a few minutes later, he was in his bed.

"I thought at first you must have done it, Mrs. Sobol," she said, turning to look at Ken.

Before I could correct her, he spoke up.

"No, I did it by myself!"

Amazing. Progress.

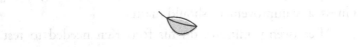

CHAPTER 22

The first hint of trouble came yesterday, just nine days after the move. As soon as I walked in the door, Miriam told me that at lunch Ken kept trying to reach across the table to poach food from his tablemates. When a staff member intervened, he began tossing his silverware across the room. Up to now, he had accepted the puréed food without question, but the sight and smell of real meat and vegetables on the other clients' plates probably was becoming too much to bear.

John and I visited the next day. The doctor had doubled the Seroquel and the morning had gone well. Ken had eaten his breakfast in the dining room with no trouble. I would have to learn to take it one day at a time. Overall it had been a good move to accept a placement here.

In the early eighties, before Ken and I started writing together, I had studied painting for a few years. I had reached the stage of entering my canvases in juried shows and selling them from time to time when a diagnosis of degenerative disc disease in my upper back put an end to painting—at least in any major way—though I continued to enjoy drawing. John, who has always been a supporter of my art, brought in three of my canvases from that time to brighten up Ken's room: a still life, a Montreal cityscape, and an abstract of our country place. While he set about hanging these, I took out a banner from a public art project Ken and I had worked on together and tacked it up. With all the added color, his room was starting to look lived in. It was time now for an excursion into the larger world.

As the three of us sat sunning ourselves in the building's front court-yard, Ken didn't comment on the change of location, but he slowly craned his head to take in the scene: ornamental shrubs in bloom, sky a pale blue, a car moving past the brick houses on the street. The sound of traffic reached us, as well as a waft of hot smoked meat from the delicatessen down the street—just as well he didn't notice that.

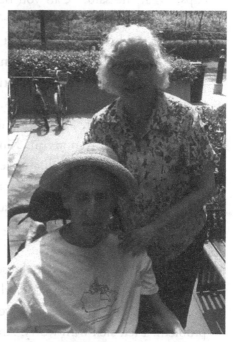

The courtyard of Kensington Gardens long-term care facility, July 22, 2010: Ken's first outing in many weeks; he enjoyed the ice cream.

Unless you count being ferried back and forth across the city by ambulance while lying flat on your back, this was his first outing of any kind in many weeks. He glanced around again, trying to take it all in. After a while, he said, very softly, "I know I'm going to have to get used to living here."

Did he really say that? John and I looked at each other.

The dietician had given us a dispensation for occasional servings of ice cream, and this seemed like the right occasion. John went in search of a treat. He returned carrying a small paper bag. "I found an old-timey store that stocks Dixie cups, Dad," he said. "Can you believe that? They even had those little wooden spoons." Dixie Cups had shrunk since my youth, or maybe it was just that at our upscale neighborhood ice cream emporium you could make a meal of one of their "small" cones. Ken finished his tiny cup quickly and John went back to the store for seconds.

A few days later, Jane and William, along with six-year-old Ximena, paid Ken a visit. Ximena had a gift for him: a large school photo on which she had carefully signed her name and written, "I love you, Grandpa," and which her parents had matted and framed. "Grandpa was in a wheelchair," she told me later. "I sat on his lap. I gave him a big hug."

Less than a week later, Ken loosened the restraints on his wheelchair, tried to get up, and fell. The doctor checked him over and said he was fine. But would falling be an ongoing problem? I felt sick with worry. And when I asked Ken about the fall, he said, "It wasn't an accident. I don't want to live through another winter."

The next time I visited, the staff had his wheelchair parked next to the nurses' desk. He had taken a turn for the worse. His eyes were closed, his body slumped forward. Miriam said they had increased the Seroquel again. And there was another new problem. "He has so much mucus in his mouth that it interferes with his eating," Miriam said. "We've been using suction on him, but he's not cooperative: He doesn't like it at all." She went to retrieve the suction gadget. This time, he opened his mouth willingly. I was glad of that; it had to feel good to have your mouth cleaned of all that gunk. I pushed the wheelchair back to his room where he quickly fell sound asleep.

Then came increased problems with his food intake. One night he had a few bites at supper; the next day he wasn't eating anything. By that evening, when I phoned to ask how he was doing, the attendant reported that his blood pressure was low and his oxygen "down a bit."

"But he's not in distress," the attendant added.

How to interpret these phrases? The changes were coming so rapidly that I couldn't really absorb them. I needed a pair of anti-gravity boots to get through the rest of the day. The increasing seriousness of his condition day by day was adding invisible weights to my body; I felt their pull down to my fingertips.

One morning in late July, I arrived to find Miriam at his bedside, looking down at him. "He's not eating," she said. I stood beside her as she momentarily studied him before turning and heading quickly out the door. She was soon back with a dish of vanilla pudding. The staff had noticed his love of sweets. He finished the few spoonfuls quickly. When he seemed to nod yes to her "more?" she hurried out again. Cavities weren't a concern now. This time, on her return, she carried a dish of ice cream, which went over even better.

So kind, I thought. Miriam is an experienced nurse; she has probably helped many families through scenes like this, yet she has never lost a bit of her humanity. In her sympathetic presence I didn't feel the usual need to apologize for tears. I confided to her my strong doubts about being able to attend the performance of an opera for which John had written the libretto; the out-of-town opening night was scheduled for next week.

Miriam urged me to go. "We're watching him carefully," she reassured me. "This afternoon, the hospital is sending over someone to make sure he's not getting dehydrated. It's a simple procedure: a needle inserted into the stomach."

By that evening, I'd had one piece of good news: Ken shows no sign of dehydration.

August 3: Although Ken was "fairly alert" yesterday (medical speak for "not unconscious/dead"?), the doctor phoned me to talk frankly about Seroquel's potential side effects. These were many: low blood pressure, heart problems, lipids, increased PD, blood sugar. I expressed my concern. The dosage was reduced.

This morning, his eyes were open—a welcome change—but his face was flushed and he was still not talking. The thermometer registered a slight fever: 38 degrees Celsius.

August 4: Ken has been placed on oxygen. I recalled the relief I felt, during an acute asthma attack, when the E.R. nurse placed a mask over my face and I could once again draw breath. I hoped Ken was feeling the same kind of comfort. His chest looked so sunken, though, one strap of his undershirt falling off his bare shoulder.

I had a date to meet a friend for lunch, but couldn't face a crowd of people. Over a table in her back yard, I spoke hopefully about the situation, the way you do to convince yourself against all hope.

August 5: I awoke around three this morning, and then kept waking at one-hour intervals. When I arrived on Ken's floor, I found the door to his room closed. I opened it, and Corry was there. She enveloped me in a hug and said she and Jane were going to phone me, but decided one of them should come in person to tell me the news. "Dad died—just minutes ago."

Jane walked in, crying. She had been here since seven a.m., she told me. "Dad was asleep at first," she said. "He seemed comfortable. I could hear him breathing. But then after awhile his breathing was so quiet that I got up and felt his chest, but I wasn't sure. By then Corry had arrived and she went to get Miriam. Miriam tried his pulse, then went to get the doctor."

"I'm just so glad he wasn't alone," I said to Jane, hugging her.

We had known for a while now that there would be no neighborhood excursions for Ken, no walking on his own, no family parties. This disease had, from the beginning, moved by stealth: long plateaus interrupted by sudden lurches. *But was he really gone?* Looking at his still form, I knew it was true, but I hadn't yet completely registered the fact. *Isn't that what people always say?*

The morning passed somehow. At some point, Miriam came in and said how sorry the staff all were. "You can stay with him as long as you like," she said, wrapping each of us in turn in an embrace. She and Marta brought tea and were kind in other small ways, all so welcome.

The chaplain stopped by. After Corry and Jane explained to him that they had to go out to make some phone calls, he turned to look at me. "I know that yours is not a religious family, Mrs. Sobol," he began. "But I just want to offer you my sympathy." I thanked him, and we made small talk. After the chaplain left, it was the coroner's turn. He was brisk and to the point, like coroners in every film I had ever seen. He signed the death certificate, offered his quick condolences, and was out the door.

I was glad to be alone with Ken for a moment. After years of anticipatory mourning and all the tears I had shed during them, by this morning I was so drained of emotion that I still hadn't cried.

The room was getting cold. I walked over to the bed to look at Ken. He no longer had need of bed covers, but instinctively I picked up the neatly folder quilt at the foot of the bed—the same colorful quilt he had carried over his arm the time he went wandering—and laid it over his body. The homey artifact helped soften the fact of death. When I leaned down to kiss him, his forehead was already cool to the touch.

The girls returned to report that they had reached John on a Greyhound bus en route to Toronto and given him the news. The three of us headed out into the lounge to make the plans that needed to be made.

CHAPTER 23

A couple of weeks after Ken's death, I walked with our children and grandchildren along a shaded pathway in the Toronto Necropolis, the city's oldest cemetery. The tall canopy that shades the grounds, an urban echo of the fields, trees, and country lanes Ken and I had never stopped missing, has been growing here for decades. John carried the urn that held Ken's ashes. An attendant discreetly followed a few steps behind, a leather bag over one shoulder.

In front of an arrangement of flowerbeds where two stone cairns stood like anchors, a small patch of earth had been freshly turned over. I glanced at the attendant. A nod of the head confirmed that, yes, this was indeed the scattering garden. Reaching into her bag, she handed me a small trowel, and stepped aside.

John held the urn as I dipped into it and transferred a

share of what was once a husband, father, father-in-law, and grandfather into the prepared spot. The action felt strange—*Are these ashes Ken?*—but not inappropriate. Cremation seems as good a way as any to deal with the death of someone you love—certainly preferable, in my opinion, to encasing them in an ornate, satin-lined box, covering it with six feet of earth, and topping the whole thing off with a forbidding-looking "rest in peace" slab of granite. (My own preference would be one that used to be followed—perhaps still is—by some North American native people, whereby the body is carefully hoisted onto a raised pallet of branches and left to weather with the seasons until nothing but the bones and teeth remain.)

One by one, everyone took their turn, until finally only eighteen-month-old Lara was left. William picked her up and helped her scoop out a small share of the ashes so she could be told, when we reminisce in future years, that she was part of this private happening on this beautiful spot during this late summer day. The attendant waited until Lara finished her assignment—grownups are always asking you to do strange things—and then handed me a small rake. We took turns smoothing the earth and laying down the white roses Corry had brought for the occasion.

We formed a semi-circle around the site for a moment of communal silence. The grandchildren glanced around, waiting to see what would happen next. Looking across at their serious faces, I felt it important to say a few words.

"I want you kids to remember something," I began. "Something that you probably already know but—but I just want to remind you of it at this time. Never forget that

Grandpa loved each and every one of you very much." They looked as though they were listening.

We stirred ourselves to leave.

The next day we held a wake of sorts at an art gallery down-town. A roomful of people watched a slide show of photos going back to Ken's childhood, shared some good laughter and a few tears, heard affectionate testimonials, listened to music, ate food. I had been worried about handling myself, but the truth was that my reaction to Ken's death had been a mixture of sadness and relief. It was only hearing Liam Clancy's baritone in the background during the slide show where I briefly lost it. Corry reached over and took my hand.

By the time Jane, Annie, Sophie, Ximena, and I joined Corry in a vocal rendition of "I'll Fly Away" from *Brother, Where Art Thou,* a favorite film of Ken's, I looked out across the crowd of relatives, old acquaintances from New York and Montreal, Parkinson's choir people, and younger people who were friends of our kids (and who had become our friends), and knew I would be fine.

Two Americans and two Canadians spoke—appropriate since Ken had lived half his life on one side of the border, half on the other. Rick Arnold started the eulogies off with a story about one of his many failed attempts to argue Ken into becoming a believer:

"Didn't it ever happen," Rick had asked Ken, "maybe when you were a kid, that you prayed for something and your prayer was answered?"

"Well, sort of," Ken had replied. "Something like that happened. But it didn't make me change my mind."

"Why not?"

"Because I didn't like the *manner* in which it was answered."

Jane Musante, the old friend to whom I had written during Ken's struggles, described her arrival at Oberlin from Charleston, West Virginia, and her encounter with a fellow freshman—a northerner who seemed to have opinions about everything. Another old friend described how, shortly after their first meeting, Ken announced that he had just formulated two life decisions: he was going to become a writer and he was going to marry me. Yet another spoke of the party-central boarding house days in London, England where he met Ken.

When John invited further comments from the crowd, one of several mourners who had been colleagues at TVO stood up and said, "When I first was introduced to Ken Sobol, I was terrified. But then one day I realized that as long as I took my job seriously, he wasn't scary at all..." That had been a typical reaction over the years among the many who had worked with Ken. Put off at first by his unusual, edgy personality, they were quickly won over by his professionalism on the job and his quirky sense of humor.

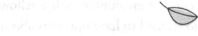

CHAPTER 24

In the days after the ceremony, the sense of Ken's still being around was strong enough that, for the first time, I understood why people sometimes keep one room exactly as it was the day the deceased "went away." I kept turning to him to tell him what a great party he had missed and expecting to hear his disbelieving reaction to the various warm testimonials. Skeptic though I am, I could even entertain the idea that maybe the line between life and death isn't as solid as we would believe. Maybe a few psychic Ken-particles continue to float around in the house's atmosphere for a while before drifting away into the ether. Who can say?

In India, if BBC documentaries are to be relied upon, there are places called "dying rooms," a tradition that reflects the idea that the end of life and the beginning of mourning intermingle as points on the same continuum. Family members may set up camp in the room, cooking special meals for the dying person as they reminisce, meditate, chant, perhaps wander over to speak with other families sharing the same space. After the dying person's final breath is drawn, the family bathes and perfumes the body and dresses it in fine robes. I liked that idea. The closest thing we have to a dying room in North America is the hospice and unfortunately, by the time Ken was eligible, there was no point in moving him to one.

After my father's funeral in 1981, a helpful older relative had made me feel better by telling me that I would make peace with his death in my own time. "Don't try to rush things, Julie," she had said. "We all of us mourn in our own way."

But my father's was a "good death;" despite his considerable discomfort from lung cancer, he was able to talk with a faraway brother over the phone, enjoy visits with grandchildren, chat with old acquaintance from his days in local politics.

A death from advanced dementia means you don't get the kind of resolution that a real good-bye brings. Verbal communication is so compromised, and has been for so long, that your thoughts and feelings are conveyed mostly through the touch of your hand or the mere fact of your presence. I didn't know how to grieve such a strange death, where the end of life and the drawn-out progressive illness that preceded it were so entangled in the mind.

Not long after the memorial service, I came across a quote from *The Shadow Box*, written by Michael Christofer, which resonated strongly: "To be bereaved is to be robbed. We do not let go willingly. Hanging onto the anger is a kind of protective covering in itself—a bulwark against the flood of sadness we fear might overwhelm us."

That was it, I decided. I had been robbed—of my best friend, my confidante, my advocate, my conversational sparring partner, my co-parent and co-grandparent. (I can teach the youngest generation many songs, but not how to hit a home run). Robbed of my carrier of heavy grocery bags, of my nightly-knightly washer-up of the supper dishes, and of my co-archivist. (No other person on the planet would be able to remember what floor we lived on in our first apartment—the fifth—or the name of the superintendent in that building—Idalberto Ray.) Even with the head start provided by years of anticipatory mourning, that was a lot of "letting go" to get through.

Our youngest daughter had always been drawn to Latin American culture (her husband, William, is Mexican) and her interest in Ingrid Betancourt, the Colombian politician who was held captive in the jungle for six years by rebel guerillas, had drawn me in. Since Betancourt's rescue in 2008, she had written a book about the experience and I had listened to interviews in which she spoke with quiet passion about her eventual forgiveness of her captors. The forgiveness can't have come easily to her; while she was enduring forced hikes on jungle trails and living on scant rations, her children had celebrated six birthdays without their mother.

Her stoicism set me wondering as to how I was doing at leaving behind the disease that had held our family captive for so long. I didn't have an easy answer, but a remark of eighteenth-century philosopher Joseph Addison was applicable:

"If suffering alone taught, all the world would be wise, since everyone suffers. To suffer must be added mourning." And mourning, I was coming to realize, is like childbirth. The fact that it is a natural process doesn't mean it comes easily; it requires your active participation. Getting rid of the protective covering against the sadness that is always waiting to overwhelm us is hard work.

Later, in October, I attended a third memorial, one organized by the staff at Kensington to honor the twelve residents who had died over the last few months. There were roses again—red ones this time—and a deeply felt sense of shared sadness in the room. The family ceremony under the trees at the Necropolis had been a last personal good-bye, the final private acknowledgment of loss after a lengthy, debilitating illness; the wake at the art gallery was a joyful celebration of Ken's life. However, this brief service at the place where he spent his last days, was something different. There was poignancy in the way the ceremony brought back memories of Ken's illness—memories that intermingled with the eleven other faces in the photos on display.

The relatives, staff, and scattering of residents seated on the metal chairs were grieving not just the death of the former residents, but also the manner of their passing. (I spotted Goodwill, one of Ken's former tablemates, in the crowd. I waved but he didn't respond.) Several among the deceased were, like Ken, dementia sufferers; all were too ill to finish their lives in the familiar comfort of their own homes.

"Ken Sobol."

Hearing his name called out, I walked to the front and

laid his rose on top of the table's growing pile of red. That part of the ceremony finished, the chaplain invited us to participate in a responsive reading.

"From the rising of the sun and in its going down…" the chaplain intoned.

We responded: "We remember them." The reading continued through a long series of call-and-response pledges.

People take oaths when they get married, when they become citizens, when they are called on to testify in court, and basically whenever the truth matters. Though nothing legal bound me to the simple promises I had just made, it felt good to speak them out loud, in front of other witnesses.

I wanted to remember Ken at these times and others.

CHAPTER 25

Remembering: the past occupies so much of our thought, dominates so much of our conversation. People speak often of their childhood memories of summer fun, adolescent adventures, past triumphs and failures, current annoyances.

We don't know the future and the present is fleeting. But we know the past because it has *passed*; it's our raw material, our life manual of instructions for thinking about the direction of our lives. People whose careers involve envisioning the future—city planners, inventors, politicians, military bigwigs, artists—spend a lot of time reviewing and rethinking the past before they come up with their visionary schemes.

I have a problem with my own rethinking, though—a sort of selective amnesia. You wouldn't think it would be difficult, given the ratio of four pre-illness decades to a single decade of illness, to recall Ken as he was in the days when he was healthy and full of opinions and enthusiasm. But ten years is a long time. The static interference from his mood shifts, paranoia, constant hallucinations, and apathy, especially during the last few months, has had a serious deprogramming effect on my ability to connect with the past.

I once read a short story about a university student who takes a summer job as a traveling photographer in rural Ontario. Many farm families, to his surprise, not only buy photos, but ask him to return the next summer. Pulling up to a familiar-looking farmhouse the following year, the young man is startled when the front door flies open and an older man rushes out to greet him emotionally. The man's only son had died suddenly, he explains, not long after the photographer's previous visit. Over the last year the farmer has tortured himself over his penny-pinching reluctance to purchase the family photos. Worst of all, lately he is starting to forget his son's face.

"If only I had that picture to look at," he laments. The photographer, seeing his despair, tells him he has kept the negatives. He will print out the photos free of charge and put them in the mail.

These days we have whole scrapbooks—or computer memory sticks—of images to help us pole vault our way back across the decades. Every once in a while, I take one of my albums down from the shelf and look through it. Whenever I get the whim, I can look at the photo of Ken and me on a Central Park bench, a baby in my arms, both of us smiling into the sunlight. (An entrepreneurial teenager was offering candid photos with his fancy new Polaroid at a dollar a shot.) Or here is one of Ken demonstrating his karate kick to my cousin Bob, a resident in one of the hippie canyons of Los Angeles. And here are the five of us on the steps to our cottage on the Bay of Fundy, Corry the same height as John before he hit his growth spurt. I look through other smiling shots of us on summer lawns in Los Angeles, Toronto, Montreal, and rural Ontario.

Even with the help of photographs, of course, memories can be fuzzy around the edges. That photo of the two of us on a pier… Was it taken out on windblown Digby Neck or at the annual scallop-shucking contest in town? Not that such details matter much in the end; these images begin to prompt other kinds of images, ones that don't need a photographic record. The song "Serenade in Blue" in a darkened lounge. The bus ride from Oberlin to Cleveland to meet Ken's parents, and late nights on the TV room's creaky leather sofa after the rest of the family was in bed. The long subway ride back and forth between his scruffy student apartment near Columbia and the downtown brownstone where I lived with Jane. Bowls of sinus-busting hot-and-sour soup at Mang Chang on Seventh Avenue, the only restaurant meal we could afford in those frugal days. The friendly rabbi flashing an encouraging smile when a combined attack of hay fever and nerves got to me during our wedding ceremony at Detroit's Temple Israel. The light-hearted mood at the reception that followed on my family's lawn, egg-salad sandwiches and lemonade catered by the ladies of the Garden City Presbyterian Church. The day had been a gift to our parents, and a final farewell to religion on our parts.

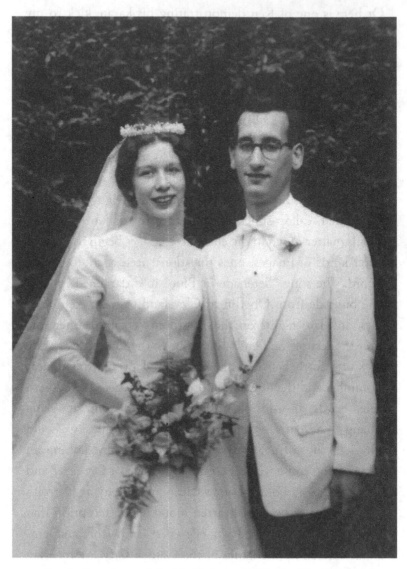

On the front lawn of the Macfie home in Garden City, Michigan,
August 1960: "The day was a gift to our parents."

For the occasion a cousin had written a rather nicely done sonnet for us. The closing couplet goes:

Let Earth with symbols of your love abound,
And thus your sep'rate, scowling priests confound.

We had done our best to bring his lines to fruition.

In April, 2011 I pay a solo visit to the Necropolis. It has been a cold spring. The trees and shrubs are at least a week behind last year's bloom. Because today is both Easter and Passover, not many people are around. At the scattering garden, I re-read Ken's plaque mounted on one of the cairns. There's a limit to what you can say in a couple of lines and I had chosen simply "Ken Sobol 1938–2010" above the five words "writer, husband, father, grandfather, friend."

I could, it now occurs to me, have added a sixth word: LBD patient. Though I didn't want those difficult years to crowd out memories of happier times, I also didn't want to lose hold of the recent past. During the last ten years, our two youngest granddaughters, Ximena and Lara, were born. Photos of them with Ken, and many shots of happy events with the other grandchildren, Ken's expression becoming increasingly befuddled with time, are dear to me in their own way—as are even the ones of him in a wheelchair during those last awful weeks. These scenes remind me that, though our caregiving was not perfect, as a family we did all we could to spare him pain. That realization is also comforting.

Coming out of my reverie, I walk slowly past the other plaques. These are the people with whom Ken, or at least part of him, is sharing eternity. It only seems appropriate to get to know more about them. I read through a number of the messages on the plaques. Most are straightforward:

Unforgettable.

She loved.

He was a gentle man.

A kind-hearted grandfather.

A good friend and neighbor.

Others offer a bit more, an intriguing glimpse into some specific aspect of the person's life:

Riding the rails in heaven.

John, beloved partner of Andrew.

D-Day, B company.

Remembering the good times with our uncle and his dogs.

Crosswords, puzzles, mysteries and knitting.

The deities that I adore/Are social peace and plenty

         —Robert Burns

Each of these distillations of lives lived strikes me with the force of poetry, but Ken would (like me) be pleased to see a great poet being put to use in this beautiful corner of our adopted city. Burns can always be counted on for a good turn of phrase.

Continuing on to the other side of the cairn, I come upon two plaques that could have been written for Ken, and which, read together, express my feelings at this quiet, private moment:

Out of pain

Peace at last, Dad.

CHAPTER 26

The wish that Ken was still here to grow old along with me is present always. In the months after the memorial, any TV drama or news report in which everything hangs on a thread—some complex escape plan or life-or-death surgery or tricky resolution of any kind—transports me back to August 5 and brings unexpected tears.

Just weeks after his death, I, along with a million or so other viewers worldwide, had watched the amazing, unexpected rescue of thirty-three Chilean miners from what seemed like certain death thousands of feet below the Atacama Desert. As each dazed, beaming man emerged blinking into the sunlight, I felt a rush of joy for his waiting family, tempered quickly by the reminder that Ken will never get that second chance at life. Our family won't be exchanging reminiscences with him about events that took place during the long siege; he and I won't have the chance to look back over our lives and clear up old misunderstandings, or perhaps start one more project together.

But you move on, sometimes without even realizing it. As the months passed I began having occasional good days when I realized, with surprise, that I was coping. Bad days were bad, but in learning to wait them out you acquired patience.

Writing helps. I wanted to get it all down, and to get it right. There is something relaxing about the simple act of nailing down a chronology, especially when trying to describe a progressive disease, where time itself is such a large part of the story. As I type, I gain a better sense of how much denial and displacement had sometimes affected me during a difficult period.

If I wake in a dismal swamp mood, I recall the advice quoted to neophyte writers looking for a way to get started: "First, apply seat of pants on seat of chair." Though I've seen the remark attributed to Ernest Hemingway, among others, literary historians trace its first use to an obscure labor organizer and novelist by the name of Mary Heaton Vorse. My own variation, directed at myself, is: "Apply soles of feet to boards of floor." Not the same level of wit, perhaps, but the point is that once you dislodge yourself from under the covers, life begins to look possible. Then you can move on to the job of applying seat of jeans to seat of computer chair.

Music helps—the reassuring, always-there keyboard, the technical challenge of a Bach prelude, the progression of chords in a Gershwin melody. The words of my early piano teachers return unbidden and their lessons make more sense to me now. I also derive enormous pleasure from the infinitely expanding jukebox known as YouTube, where I can call up any version of any piece of music I have ever enjoyed and then read through other listeners' impassioned opinions about the performance; I had no idea so many people felt that vehemently about every musician from Caruso to Glenn Gould and on to Walk Off the Earth and beyond.

Meanwhile, the youngest generation drags me, not all that unwilling, farther and farther into the future. A disc compiled by Elliot, Corry and Greg's younger son, enables me to tell White Stripes from Foo Fighters and Blackeyed Peas. John has set me up with a Facebook page, and I am pleased when fourteen-year-old Louis writes encouragingly: "YOU GOT FACEBOOK!?! Awesome, grandma, welcome aboard."

In real time, away from Facebook, I am supported by old friends who know where I'm coming from and new friends familiar with my recent past. Among the latter are two neighbors with first-hand experience of LBD. Fiona's husband died days after Ken; Joyce's husband has for several years been in a care facility where she visits him every day. My only regret is that we learned of each other's existence only days before Ken's death. Though the details of our stories vary, the timelines are similar, from the puzzling early signs and the challenge of finding a diagnosis to the mysterious visions, the crisis, and the eventual move into care: the sadness, the love, the confusion, the self-doubt, all of it. I'm glad to have met these two, even late in the day.

My own mortality looms larger since Ken's death. The manufacturer of my battery-run wall clock included an artificial ticking noise, which brings back visits to ancient aunts and uncles in farmhouses filled with Victorian bric-a-brac and where an old pendulum clock counted the moments off, one-by-one by tick-tock one.

As a self-obsessed teenager I used to enjoy brooding on my own death, veering back and forth between Dostoevskian discomfort at the very notion of it on one hand and the insouciant attitude of World War I poets like Alan Seeger on the other. In the latter mood I used to recite "I Have a Rendezvous With Death" to myself as I waited for the inter-urban bus to carry me to my weekly piano lesson.

That teenage ambivalence returns at times, mostly on days when chronic aches and pains join forces to weaken my resolve; but mostly I've come to accept that death is a part of life. Or, at least I can say I believe that we have it in ourselves to face death with a degree of equanimity—perhaps even, at a certain point, with open arms.

In the meantime, living well is still the best revenge.

AFTERWORD

My Eight Suggestions for Health Care Professionals

1. Understand how much early detection matters to people with LBD *and to their families.* Toward that end, make better use of what's out there: sleep tests, personality surveys, polysomnograms, visual-spatial tests, blood tests (to rule out other causes), CTs and MRIs (to detect brain shrinkage), ECGs (with a careful look at Q-T intervals), dopamine transporter imaging, and Structural Abnormality Index.

2. Include family members as an active part of the medical team. Doctors contribute professional expertise, but family caregivers can provide background and daily first-hand insight into the ever-changing symptoms. Both types of information are needed.

3. Upon diagnosis, whether you're a family doctor, geriatrician, neurologist, or psychiatrist, provide families
   with informational brochures and a list of useful websites and agencies. (A simple step, and one already
   followed by specialists in other diseases.)

4. Follow the path already set by Korea, Australia,
   Norway, the Netherlands, France, Scotland, and the
   United Kingdom. In South Korea, where the dementia population is expected to grow from 7 percent in
   2000 to 14 percent in 2018 to 20 percent (!) in 2026,
   long-term care insurance is paid through national
   health insurance premiums. The president of the
   Korean Alzheimer's Association conducts seminars
   on self-esteem for patients and gives talks to everyone from nursing home staff to bus drivers and bank
   tellers: The Ministry of Knowledge Economy runs a
   "comprehensive experience hall" to deal with dementia. Teenagers receive credit for visiting nursing homes
   and giving foot massages. Grade school kids study the
   brain, with a chunk of tofu standing in for the real
   thing.

5. Invite caregivers and early-stage LBD patients to give
   joint talks at care facilities, hospitals, and community
   centers. Also, offer more dementia seminars in medical and nursing schools, and in social work programs.

6. Set up LBD websites in every language. Dementia is a
   universal affliction.

7. Advocate for tax breaks for caregivers in recognition of their unpaid round-the-clock work. Some families lose two incomes: the patient's and the caregiver's.

8. Consider rebranding Lewy Body Dementia as "Kosaka's Disease" after LBD researcher Dr. Kenji Kosaka. That way no one would have to waste time repeatedly explaining the odd-sounding name now in use. ("How do you spell it? What is a lueyboddy anyway?")

Beyond these simple, practical steps, as the world's population ages more frank discussion of larger end-of-life issues, from intubation to pain relief to diet to DNR requests, is needed.

FURTHER READING

Books

Baird, Jean and George Bowering, *The Heart Does Break: Canadian Writers on Grief and Mourning* (Toronto: Vintage Canada, 2011).

Bertman, Sandra L., *Facing Death: Images, Insights, and Interventions* (New York: Brunner-Routledge, 1991).

Ginsburg, Lidiia, translated by Alan Myers, *Blockade Diary* (UK: Random House, 1998).

Kitwood, Tom, *Dementia Reconsidered: The Person Comes First* (UK: Open University Press, 1997).

Mace, Nancy L. and Peter V. Rabins, *The 36-Hour Day: A*

Family Guide to Caring for Persons with Alzheimer Disease, Related Dementing Illnesses, and Memory Loss in Later Life Warner Books, revised edition 2001).

Payne, Christopher and Sachs, Oliver, *Asylum: Inside the Closed World of State Mental Hospitals* (USA: MIT Press, 2009).

Shulman, Alix Kates, *To Love What Is: A Marriage Transformed* (New York: Farrar, Straus & Giroux, 2008).

Tomkins, Calvin, *Living Well is the Best Revenge* (New York: Modern Library, 1998).

Articles

Alzheimer Society of Canada, *Rising Tide: The Impact of Dementia on Canadian Society*, Alzheimer Society of Canada, Toronto, 2010.

Aviv, Rachel, "God Knows Where I Am: What Should Happen When Patients Reject Their Diagnosis," *The New Yorker*, May 30, 2011.

Belluck, Pam, "Children Ease Alzheimer's in Land of Aging," *The New York Times*, November 26, 2010.

Bostrom, Fredrik, MD (with Linus Jonsson MD, Lennart Minthon MD, Elisabet London MD), "Quality of Life in Dementia With Lewy Bodies," *International Journal of Geriatric Psychiatry* 21, no. 12 (December 2006).

Brain Repair Centre, "Study will provide snapshot of what it's like to live with a neurological disorder," in *Brainwaves*, Dalhousie University, February 2012, http://www. brainrepair.ca/images/pdf/2012-02-Enewsletter.pdf

Dementia, http://www.wikipedia.org

Galvin, James E., MD (with H. Malcom, D. Johnson, J. C. Morris MD), "Personality Changes May Help Detect Form of Dementia," *Neurology*, Washington University School of Medicine, May 29, 2007, http://neuro-wustl.edu/ news/enewsletter/

Gawande, Dr. Atul, "Letting Go," *The New Yorker*, August 2, 2010.

Hauw, J. J., MD (with C. Hausser-Hauw MD, U. De Girolami MD, D. Hasboun MD, D. Seilhean MD), "Neuropathology of Sleep Disorders: A Review," *Journal of Neuropathology and Experimental Neurology* 70, no. 4 (April 2011): 242–252.

Kahn, Andrew, "Writer's Blockade," *Times Literary Supplement*, September 9, 2011 (article about Lidiya Ginzburg).

Learn.Genetics, "Prions: On the Trail of Killer Proteins," University of Utah (a cogent online summary provided for classroom use), http://learn.genetics.utah.edu/ content/begin/dna/prions

Leverenz, James, MD, and Andrew David, "Confronting a Century of Lewy Body Confusion," *Dimensions*, An Aging & Alzheimer's Update, University of Washington Alzheimer's Disease Research Center, Spring 2011.

Mehta, Aalok, "Protein Folding: A New Twist on Brain Disease", BrainFacts.org, May 16, 2010, http://www.brainfacts.org/diseases-disorders/ degenerative-disorders/articles/2010

Mehta, Aalok, "Alzheimer's Disease and Dementia Today" BrainFacts.org, February 14, 2012, http://www.brainfacts. org/diseases-disorders/degenerative-disorders/articles/2012/ alzheimers-disease-today/

Nunez, Rafael E. and Eve Sweetser "With the Future Behind Them: Convergent Evidence from Aymara Language and Gesture in the Crosslinguistic Comparison of Spatial Construals of Time," *Cognitive Science* 30 (2006): 1–49.

Rose, Charlie, "The Brain Series," http://www.charleyrose.com

Silin, Peter S., "Moving into a Nursing Home: A Guide for Families," The Caregiver's Beacon (online newsletter), March 1, 2011, http://www.ec-online.net/ knowledge/articles/ nursinghomemove.html

Smith, Amanda G., MD, "Behavioral Problems in Dementia," *Postgraduate Medicine* 115, no. 6 (June 2004).

Strobel, Gabrielle, *Neither Fish Nor Fowl: Dementia with Lewy Bodies Often Missed*, Alzheimer Research Forum, June 2009, http://www.alzforum.org

Valeo, Tom, "The Other Dementias," *Neurology Now* 5 no. 6, (Nov./Dec. 2009): 26–27,31–34.

Brochures and information sheets available from the Parkinson Society and the Alzheimer Society in your city.

ACKNOWLEDGMENTS

My thanks to the people who took the time to read and comment on this book at various stages in its development: Meg Masters, Ellen Moore, Dr. Alastair Flint, Dr. Anh Nguyen, Zoe Levitt, Caroline Bady, David Bady, Julian Clarke, John Sobol, and Corry Sobol.

The enthusiasm for the project expressed from the beginning by my friends Pat Derbacz, Joyce McClelland, Fiona McHugh, and Larry Levy helped keep me going as I moved on to the later chapters.

In addition to social worker Zoe Levitt at Toronto General Hospital, Jean Noguira (St. Christopher House) Sheila Katz (Toronto Western Hospital) and Jennifer Kivell (the Alzheimer's Society of Toronto) provided essential information, sympathy, and practical suggestions during a difficult time.

To Dr. Flint, Dr. Nguyen, Dr. A. Birnbaum, and Dr. Gordon Hardacre, I express my appreciation for their concern about Ken's wellbeing and for their wealth of medical expertise.

At Second Story Press I benefited from the comradely support of Carolyn Jackson and Margie Wolfe. Thanks also to Nadiya Osmani for her hard work on the project.

My family, such an integral part of this book's story, also encouraged me in the writing of it. This has meant a lot to me, and I thank each of them warmly for their support.

Finally, I want to thank John Paul Lathers for the quote from his "Sonnet for August 28," and to commend the unsung heroes who volunteer their time at the following websites: the Lewy Body Dementia Association in the U.S. (www.lewybodydementia.org) and the Lewy Body Society in the U.K. (www.lewybody.org).

ABOUT THE AUTHORS

Julie Macfie Sobol and Ken Sobol met at Ohio's Oberlin College in 1958. After marrying and living in New York, London, and Los Angeles, they and their three children moved to Canada. There Ken continued his Emmy-winning writing career with TVOntario and other networks, mainly in children's television and TV documentaries. He also authored several children's books. Julie is a painter and musician who has worked as a piano teacher and accompanist. Her paintings hang in Canada, the U.S., and England. Julie and Ken began writing together for magazines in the 1980s, and then went on to write two books of social history: *Looking for Lake Erie* and *Lake Erie: A Pictorial History*. *Love and Forgetting* began as a magazine piece about Lewy Body Dementia after Ken was diagnosed with the disease in 2007. The couple was forced to find new ways of living and writing together as

Ken's symptoms deepened, their understanding of the disease increased, and the article morphed into a book. Ken died in August of 2010, just three weeks after moving into a long-term care facility. Julie, now a grandmother of six, continues to make her home in Toronto.